CATCHING THE WORM

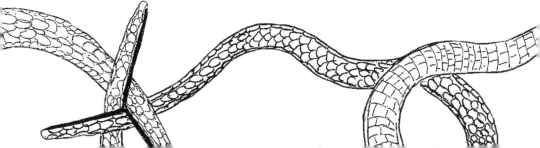

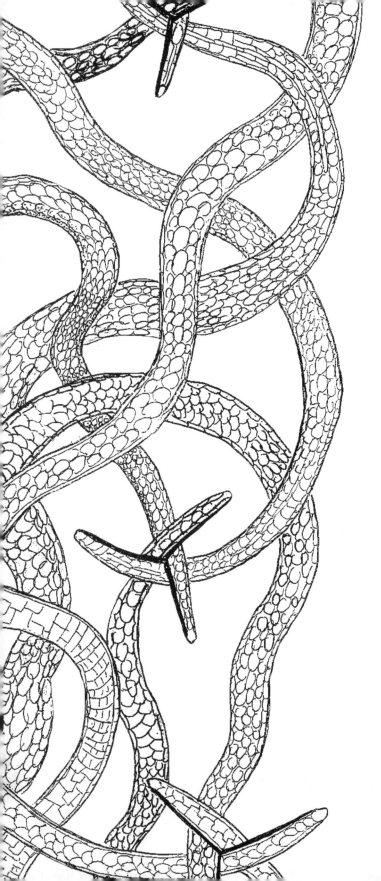

Catching
the worm

Towards ending river blindness,
and reflections on my life

WILLIAM C. CAMPBELL

with CLAIRE O'CONNELL

Catching the worm: towards ending river blindness, and reflections on my life

First published 2020
Royal Irish Academy, 19 Dawson Street, Dublin 2
www.ria.ie

'Fasciola' © 1988 Johns Hopkins University
Press. First published in *Perspectives in Biology
and Medicine* 31 (4) (Summer 1988), p. 506.
Reproduced with permission by Johns Hopkins
University Press.

'Onchocerca' © 1988 Johns Hopkins University
Press. First published in *Perspectives in Biology
and Medicine* 32 (1) (Autumn 1988), p. 108.
Reproduced with permission by Johns Hopkins
University Press.

'M&B 693' © 1990 Johns Hopkins University
Press. First published in *Perspectives in Biology
and Medicine*, 33 (3) (Spring 1990), pp 389–90.
Reproduced with permission by Johns Hopkins
University Press.

ISBN 978-1-911479-33-8 (HB)
ISBN 978-1-911479-34-5 (pdf)
ISBN 978-1-911479-35-2 (epub)
ISBN 978-1-911479-36-9 (mobi)

British Library Cataloguing in Publication Data.
A CIP catalogue record for this book is available
from the British Library.

Design: Fidelma Slattery
Editor: Helena King
Indexer: Lisa Scholey
Printed in Ireland by Watermans Printers Ltd

This publication has received support from

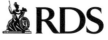

Royal Irish Academy is a member of Publishing
Ireland, the Irish book publishers' association

A NOTE FROM THE PUBLISHER

We want to try to offset the environmental impacts
of carbon produced during the production of our
books. For the production of this book we will
plant 30 trees with Easy Treesie.

The Easy Treesie – Crann Project organises children
to plant trees. The aim is to plant a tree for every
child in Ireland. A million trees by 2023. This is
inspired by and part of the Trillion Tree Campaign,
which is a project of Plant-for-the-Planet to plant
a trillion trees. This initiative is a development and
continuation of the activities of the earlier Billion
Tree Campaign, which was instigated by Nobel
Laureate Wangari Maathai, who founded the Green
Belt Movement in Africa in 1977.

Crann – 'Trees for Ireland' is a membership-based,
non-profit, registered charity (CHY13698) uniting
people with a love of trees. It was formed in 1986
by Jan Alexander, with the aim of "Releafing
Ireland". Its mission is to enhance the environment
of Ireland through planting, promoting, protecting
and increasing awareness about trees and
woodlands.

www.easytreesie.com

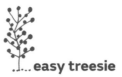

DEDICATED TO

my family and friends,
in gratitude for my life and for their enrichment
of its many years

AND TO

my brilliant colleagues at Merck & Co. Inc.
and at Drew University, with whom I was privileged to work

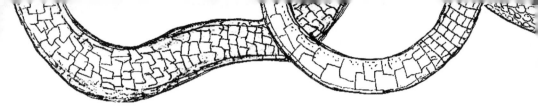

CONTENTS

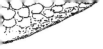
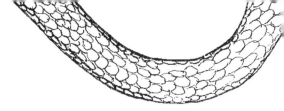

CONTENTS

A phone call
that changed everything

I wasn't expecting the phone call. I didn't even know that the Nobel prizes were being announced that day. But early on the morning of 5 October 2015, the phone rang in the house I share with my wife, Mary, in Massachusetts. The next moment, our lives changed.

I learned that I had been named as a recipient of the Nobel Prize for Physiology or Medicine for that year. The prize was shared with Professor Satoshi Ōmura and Professor Tu Youyou for our discoveries concerning therapies against parasitic diseases. For Professor Ōmura and me, that related to a new medicine—ivermectin—that is effective against the tiny worms that cause river blindness in humans.

The story of how ivermectin was discovered, how it became one of the blockbuster veterinary drugs against parasites and how ivermectin came to treat river blindness spans almost two decades. Starting in the mid-1970s, it involved more than 100 people directly on research, clinical trials and drug distribution. In 1987 Merck & Co. Inc. announced publicly that it would donate ivermectin free of charge to all patients who needed it for the treatment of river blindness. Thanks to the donation of the drug by Merck and the efforts of many dedicated agencies, the impact of that research has been huge. To date millions of people have been treated with ivermectin to avoid the disabling symptoms of river blindness, and the disease has been certified as 'eliminated' in four South American countries and has been and vastly reduced in sub-Saharan Africa. The human misery and loss that has been spared because of ivermectin is enormous.

That said, I was not in any way expecting the call that October morning. By then, I was 85 and I was well into an enjoyable retirement. The Nobel news brought me rapidly back out of it, and I soon discovered that being a Nobel laureate is not for the faint of heart. Since then, I have been kept busy, perhaps as busy as ever before.

The responses from Ireland to the news of the award were especially warm and enthusiastic—after all, it was the first time a native of Ireland had received the Nobel prize in Physiology or Medicine. Indeed, the only other Irish Nobel laureate in any of the sciences was Ernest T.S. Walton, who had been my physics lecturer at Trinity College Dublin. He shared the Nobel prize in Physics in 1951 with J.D. Cockcroft, for his part in 'splitting the atom'.

But I have struggled with the recognition of me as an individual scientist. In reality, the work that has had such an impact on river blindness in humans and on the prevention of disease in domestic animals involved a long progression of incremental steps, large teams and the wisdom of many people. To them, I am indebted, and I have felt the weight of that debt while reflecting on my almost-90-year journey: from growing up in rural Ireland to studying parasitology at Trinity College Dublin, then moving to the US to further my studies and subsequently building a career in the pharmaceutical industry.

Bringing together my memories and reflections has prompted me to think about the balance between those that might interest me, their main protagonist, and the aspects of my life that would have broader appeal. There is also the vexing question of who is gathering these stories and reflections: as I have grown older, I have slowly and imperceptibly developed a suspicion that we are, at some level, different people at different times. It is enough for me now, though, to simply hold fast to the concept of a personhood, inculcated in the mind long ago.

James Pope-Hennessy, who wrote on the life and work of the Victorian novelist Anthony Trollope, noted, unsurprisingly, that Trollope's own *Autobiography* was an 'essential source' for biographers such as himself. Initially, Hennessy found the *Autobiography* to be 'candid, artless, complacent, and truthful'. On further reading, however, he came to the conclusion that Trollope's autobiography was 'both smug and deceptive'. What he found especially frustrating was that Trollope had chosen to leave out 'an enormous amount of personal feelings and intimate events'. In contrast, in the upcoming pages I speak often of feelings and emotions.

Ramelton,
County Donegal

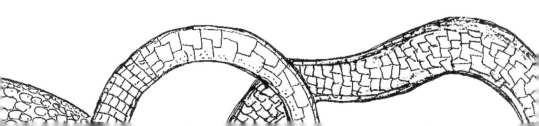

A Ramelton childhood

Our busy house was in the town of Ramelton in County Donegal, Ireland. There had been scattered early settlements in the region, but the beginning of the town itself coincided very neatly with the beginning of the seventeenth century. Though I had been born in County Derry (in Londonderry in 1930), I lived with my family in Ramelton throughout childhood and early adulthood. We lived on The Mall, in a terrace of houses by the estuary of the Lennon River, a short distance from where the waters flow into Lough Swilly and then onwards to the Atlantic Ocean. As a child, I would occasionally see boats arriving from England to disgorge their deliveries of coal. Over the years as the harbour silted up, the port traffic slowed almost to a complete stop, but the river remained the defining landmark of the town.

One of my earliest memories from childhood is learning manners in French from Mademoiselle Heckendorn, a Swiss nanny who lived with us when I was very young. To this day, I have no idea what her first name was. We called her 'Mademoiselle'. She would teach myself and my brothers Bert and Lexie phrases in French—my sister Marion was still too young—so that we could ask permission to leave the dinner table, or the classroom. *Puis-je quitter la salle s'il vous plaît? Permettez-moi a quitter la table s'il vous plaît?* We were exposed early to the cultural concept of foreign language. I have no other memory of her brief presence in our lives, and have no idea of when or why she left.

Our house was one of two that adjoined my father's shop, R.J. Campbell's. The house closer to the shop was occupied by the family of Sam Buchanan. He was manager of the four or five counter-hands who worked in the shop, leaving my father time to focus on the growth of the business, which was very successful. My father sold groceries, hardware and china, he bought and sold potatoes and grass seed for wholesale shipment and export, and he was meticulous in his dealings with the farmers. He had a black notebook and, when someone would come in looking to sell him grass seed, he would scatter some on the notebook's cover and examine them with a magnifying glass to assess the quality of that batch.

My father and mother would occasionally attend commercial shows in Dublin and order the very latest thing in household furnishings. I remember the kitchen being renovated and given a floor of solid green rubber (undoubtedly vulcanised), with black stripes inlaid in a geometric pattern. It was very modern for those days and was a conversation piece among visitors. It was a great success, yet I don't remember seeing such a floor anywhere else.

The porosity of house and shop meant there were people around all the time. At one end of the kitchen sat a long table, and the people who worked in the shop would come in for mid-morning and mid-afternoon tea. My mother and the maid would go into high gear at those times, serving hot tea and scones my mother had baked. As children, we loved to hang around the kitchen and chat with, and get teased by, the counter-hands and the shop secretary—a male, as was customary in such establishments.

Some of those table chatterers were like part of the family. One, Wee David Anderson (not to be confused with Big David Anderson, a relative and co-worker in the shop), began working at the shop when he was a teenager. He lived in a small attic bedroom in our house when he was an apprentice, and as well as having morning and afternoon tea he would also have lunch with us. Later on, he got married and didn't live with us any more—though he still ate lunch with our family and worked in the shop until he retired many decades later, leaving a proud record of never missing a day of work. My father had a similar arrangement at the start of his retail career. Before setting up his own business in Ramelton he had served as a shop apprentice in Milford, Co. Donegal, about five miles (7 km) away.

Our house and shop were busy places, inside and out. Local farmers would arrive in their cars, or even in horses and carts. That was not unusual, and occasionally even a donkey and cart arrived for the owner to pick up wares.

A big character around our business was a local man named Jamie Irwin. An unmarried man, he mostly lived by himself. He worked for my father until my father's death, then continued to work for my mother until he himself died. Jamie was remarkable. He looked after the dogs, the cows and the chickens, did all the gardening, and managed the milking. In his own arena he was very much in charge. He would walk the cows up onto a farm that my father had on high ground across the river, and he would tell us kids to get out of the way or engage us in spirited conversation as the mood struck him. He was an interesting man and on occasion, when a cow was expected to calve, he would sit up with my father and recite Burns' poetry.

As the work and commerce went on, we kids wove in and out of the shop and house, doing childhood things. I was not particularly athletic as a child, and had little interest in team sports apart from the local soccer matches. But all the boys, myself included, followed the boxing news. If Joe Louis was scheduled to fight, we would plan to sit up until the wee hours of the morning to listen to the live commentary on the 'wireless'. I have the distinct impression that, because of weakness either in our resolve or in transatlantic broadcasting, we (unlike Mr Louis) seldom succeeded in our objective.

I was the reader in our family, and like many children, I would read long past the allotted time at night. I made a flashlight using a big, squarish, flattish battery that would sit in the palm of your hand. It had two little prongs or electrodes, and I would climb under the blanket and push the battery prongs close together so as to touch them against a little lightbulb so I could illuminate my reading.

My father had a lovely bookcase built into the house. He didn't do much reading, but he liked the idea of reading and he liked having books. We had *The children's encyclopaedia* edited by Arthur Mee, and one of my most joyous memories of childhood is when my cousins visited one Christmas and gave me a present of a Biggles book, one of a series by Capt. W.E. Johns (it is funny how some names stick in memory seemingly forever). I immediately became entranced by the tales of this glamorous pilot flying in all directions, and it kindled an interest in planes that endured throughout my youth and adolescence.

In my early teenage years I spent a lot of time alone, because my brothers were at boarding-school and my sister was four years younger than I was. But I had a few childhood friends, and some of them lived very close by. The McCreas lived two doors down, and I was good friends with Basil, who was around my age. We and the other local boys played hide-and-seek, and practised shooting soccer goals and hockey goals using gateways or improvised goal-posts. We also played in the stores behind my father's shop. I sustained a life-long scar when I fell on a metal fireplace there, failing to make a jump the older boys had done. The wound bled profusely, as scalp wounds can do, and I rushed to my mother. She was appalled to see all that blood gushing from my head. I don't recall quite how she staunched the bleeding, but in our household the first-aid treatment of choice for cuts and grazes was the antiseptic tincture of iodine. It was fiercely violet in colour, and being a tincture it was alcohol-based and stung sharply on application. In fact, I suspect that much of the ordeal of sustaining a cut or a graze was the treatment afterwards, and one felt more relieved to have survived the stinging than to have survived the original trauma.

As kids, we did a lot of make-believe and acting-out stuff, and could often be found in the limbs of our favourite climbable tree—a tree that could easily become a ship or a plane. We seldom visited each others' houses, and the same could be said of the grown-ups in the community, although small adult dinner parties and children's birthday parties did occasionally occur.

The house in between our house and the McCrea house served as 'the Guards Barracks' or police station. The sergeant and his family lived on the top floor. Out at the back of the barracks there was a cell, a little concrete outbuilding where the guards could lock up the unruly. This cell was known as the black hole, and sometimes we could hear drunken people yelling from inside there in the middle of the night. The noise was never commented on the next day by the adults of the house, at least not to us children.

We were members of Ramelton Presbyterian Church. As children, we were totally unaware that it was a church of historical significance. It was the home church of Francis Makemie, who went to America in the 1680s and became one of the founders of the Presbyterian church in what would become the United

States; he went on to fight and win a major battle for separation of church and state. His old church building still stands and was featured, with Makemie himself, on an Irish stamp in 1982.

Often in public discourse, the subject of religion is best left alone. Yet despite the fervent disbelief and pleading of modern atheists, the subject does not go away. I grew to doubt the religious faith in which I was brought up, but I have never been comfortable with that doubt—or with faith. Faith in something demonstrably factual is meaningless. Indeed, faith presupposes doubt. I have been good at doubting, yet have never been able to reject religious faith. More accurately, I have been able to reject a fair amount of Christian scripture without resorting to atheism.

Modern philosophers seem to be prone to atheism. I find comfort and delight in Gabriel Dante Rossetti's remark: 'The worst moment for the atheist is when he is really thankful and has nobody to thank.' Juxtaposition of those two outlooks can perhaps be seen as a reminder that lack of religious faith on your part does not entitle you to be dismissive of the religious faith of others. In similar vein, I have always sympathised with Charles Darwin's sadness when it 'dawned' on him that his loss of faith and his knowledge of earth and sky had made him unable to find pleasure in a beautiful sunset.

The life and work of the artist Vincent van Gogh have been adequately, perhaps excessively, exposed to public scrutiny, yet one seldom comes across a reference to what I consider the most poignant moment of his life. It happened when van Gogh was in his 30s. He had become an atheist—and sufficiently doubtful about his own sanity that he had committed himself to an insane asylum. The moment of which I am speaking was recorded in a letter to his beloved brother Theo, and is recalled in Alan Lightman's *Searching for stars on an island in Maine*. Vincent said that he had a 'tremendous need for, shall I say the word—for religion—so I go outside at night to paint the stars'.

Stars are rather prominently featured in some of van Gogh's most admired paintings. What impresses me about that letter is that this man was crying out in visceral and desperate need for something awesome in his life. One could argue that his precarious mental status diminishes any significance that can be attached to his statement, but looking up at the stars on a dark night is surely an awesome thing. Profound awe surely presupposes profound mystery—mystery beyond human reach. It would seem unlikely that an all-knowing, all-powerful God would need us mere mortals—but I have no problem at all in identifying with those who feel that they need God. I have always felt that I need God. I need God to be, in the words of the songster, 'someone to watch over me'.

Then, too, I have found intellectual comfort, if not intellectual reassurance, from the records of eminent scientists (the names Carl Sagan and, again, Alan Lightman come to mind) who spurn religious faith but eventually encounter a circumstance that baffles their rationality so compellingly that they turn to something at least vaguely transcendental. They, like many others, might settle for Thomas Henry Huxley's agnosticism. In early adulthood, I took refuge there myself, and remain susceptible to its appeal.

As a child, though, I would go to Church with my family each Sunday. Sometimes, farmers who lived out of town would walk miles and miles to get to church. Or they might arrive on bicycle, or even by pony and trap. Later on, they drove their cars, causing huge congestion around the church in our little town as they looked for parking spaces. The minister of our Church, Reverend Scott, and his wife were good friends with my parents, and I suspect the Scotts influenced my parents in a way that shaped our lives. My father would have leaned on them for guidance about education and family matters, and I have no doubt that the Scotts had a hand in selecting our tutor, Miss Martin, who had a profound impact on me as one of my earliest teachers.

But at the time I was oblivious to such things. For me, growing up in Ramelton was a time of security, curiosity and bustle, darting in and out of the commerce and collegiality of business, friends and family.

Mother meets Father

Sarah Jane ('Sadie') Patterson grew up at Morroe, a cluster of three houses on farmland near Dunfanaghy, County Donegal. Her mother (Rebecca McAdoo Patterson) died at age 31, leaving her husband, Thomas, and four young children. Among the relatives and friends who were prominent in Sadie's young life was Sarah Jane Hunter, a relative close enough to be called Aunt, and who in fact became a mother-figure to Sadie.

Mrs Hunter did not live in the Dunfanaghy area but in Ramelton, and would often invite the now-grown-up Sadie to come and stay with her. Her house in Ramelton was on The Mall, and it so happened that it was just a few doors away from the home of a young man who had bought a tiny grocery store and was working hard at making a success of it. Mrs Hunter would, on occasion, invite the young man, Robert John Campbell, to dinner. Romance blossomed, and, in the course of time, Sadie and Robert John married (in 1926).

These central facts seeped into my awareness over time, but it is only now, much later, that I have come to suspect that, in the meeting of these two young people, there may have been not only an element of chance, but also a measure of beneficent social scheming.

My father, too, had grown up on a farm on Donegal's Fanad Peninsula—but in the neighbourhood of Drumfad rather than Dunfanaghy. Both of my parents were from backgrounds of Protestant farmers, a population historically common in the northern part of Donegal: plain-spoken, hardworking, abstemious people, committed to lay governance in church affairs, and occupied mostly in the raising of sheep and cattle and the harvesting of oats, barley and potatoes.

Apparently my father had not been entirely without competition. Late in life, my widowed mother received an afternoon caller, a visitor from Canada. She told me afterwards that he was a friend of long ago, who had once hoped to marry her and emigrate with her to Canada. My father, at one point, had also come close to emigrating to Canada—but that was before he met my mother.

For their honeymoon, my parents decided on the big adventure of going to the Isle of Man. The first stop on their journey was Belfast. There they got a message, presumably by telegram or phone call to their hotel, telling them Mrs Hunter was dead. The newlyweds turned back immediately for home. At some later date, my father and mother did visit the Isle of Man. In older age they made a trip to the Canary Islands. I think it was the first aeroplane flight for both of them. They were fascinated; but 'leisure travel' was not their sort of thing, and they never did it again. They were by no means unwilling to try new things, but (as was common in those days) they usually found novelty within the sphere of their daily lives.

My family in Ramelton

Soon after I moved from Ireland to the United States in my early 20s, I sent a letter to my parents; it may not have been the very first, but it was one of the first letters sent home. In it I said 'Not a day passes that I do not think often and lovingly of home.' Though I do not have a copy of the letter, I can put those words in quotation marks because I remember how extraordinary they were, in the setting of a non-demonstrative family living in a culture of reticence.

Given the time and place, the quoted words must have been received as a thunder clap—a shocking outburst of raw emotion! Years later on a visit to my Ramelton home, I looked in the drawer of the sideboard in the living room in which very special documents were kept. Sure enough, that letter was there. I have never been so thankful to have written a letter.

In it, I also thanked my parents for the opportunity to go to college, adding that there was no university other than Trinity College Dublin to which I would rather have gone. When I was a student at Trinity, my father came to visit me and took me to the movies. My older brother Lexie was no longer in College, and I think my father felt an obligation to take me to see a movie as a treat. But in the middle of it, he turned and asked me if I thought it was good. I remember (with regret) that I found his question annoying. My father wondered whether I was enjoying being at the movies, and it was very clear that he was not. This had nothing to do with the actors or the action on the silver screen: my father simply could not engage with what he saw as frivolous activities.

It was always that way. Recreation was just not something he did. He had a fishing rod hanging up in his office—perhaps someone had given it to him as a present—but it was never used. And when my brothers and I were very young, he brought us to see local soccer games a couple of times. You could pay 6 pence on entry and then stand on a bank where there was a break in the hedge to get a better view; but my father would be conspicuously miserable!

Looking back, it might be tempting to call him a workaholic, but that modern label would not fit. We lived at a latitude comparable to that of Labrador in Canada, though the Gulf Stream made our climate much milder. There was no air-conditioning. It was a region of small farms and small businesses. The vast majority of people worked long hours and worked hard. Recreation and hobbies were not common topics of conversation.

On my birth certificate, issued in 1930 when my father was in his late 40s, his profession is listed as 'grocer', and he was a gifted entrepreneur by nature. He had started in business in 1919 with a rat-infested little hole-in-the-wall shop that he bought in Ramelton, and over the years he built it up to become the largest shop in the region, with two warehouses and a lorry. It became R.J. Campbell (Donegal) Ltd. As already mentioned, my father sold anything and everything—from gramophone records to cabbages from our garden; from cups-and-saucers to plums and ploughs. Farm implements, indeed, were a specialty, and during business hours the street in front of the shop was always lined with shiny new ploughs, reapers, mechanical hay-rakes and such. Goods such as timber, glass and hardware were delivered around the countryside.

Potatoes were collected from farmers in season. For a half-year after graduating from college, in 1952, I 'was volunteered' to work part-time on the lorry. I must confess that there were times when I was unseemly conscious of the fact that nobody knew that the kid who was hauling a sack of potatoes onto the lorry had a first-class honours degree in science. My parents, of course, would have taken for granted that time on the lorry would be good for body and soul.

We had about half a dozen cows, and, from time to time my mother would make butter from their milk. When I was a child, an electric milking machine was installed in a small building at the back of our house, not far from the byre. We were the first in the region to get such a thing, and people from the company that made the machine came and installed it. We also had an electric churn, and a cream separator with its interleaved sheets of thin steel.

This kind of innovation was typical of my father and mother—we were the first in the town to get several items of modern equipment, including an Esse cooker and a refrigerator. They would do it quietly and without fuss. And, of course, there was a business side to it—when my mother used the butter churn, word would spread that fresh butter was (briefly!) available at R.J.'s.

My father electrified Ramelton, in a literal way. He was the person who brought electricity to the town: he put in the poles that carried the wires and he bought a big steam-powered generator, an impressive machine with a huge flywheel. For us kids it was pretty intimidating. It was started with compressed air, and it had to run three cycles of breaking-in every time it ran. It made a loud chuff-chuff noise, and because of this, when I was very sick with pneumonia as a child, he switched it off in case the noise was disturbing me—a thoughtful parental gesture.

My father sold the electricity that was generated: people in the town paid him per kilowatt hour used. He started before the national Electricity Supply Board was established in 1927, and records show that in 1929 he supplied 35 homes and businesses, rising to 133 by 1954.

Having the generator—first the large fly-wheeled contraption and later a diesel-fuelled setup—meant that my father controlled the electricity supply to the town. During the Second World War, when oil was severely rationed, he had to turn the power off during some daylight hours and late at night. Sometimes though, people would ask him to leave it on. A woman who lived near us on The Mall once called him and asked him to turn on the power because she was going to a special function and she needed to iron a dress. On another occasion, the Irish army was planning a big dance in the town, so they dropped off a few barrels of oil at my father's shop and asked him would he please leave the lights on. He did.

Not everyone was so blessed. In 2012, one of Reverend Scott's grown-up children, Dermot, wrote an amusing memoir piece in *The Irish Times*. He wrote that he had been born at 3 a.m., and his arrival had been illuminated by an oil lamp—because Mr Campbell had switched off the engine and gone to bed!

My father continued to provide the electricity for Ramelton—at least until his bedtime—for several years until eventually the Electricity Supply Board bought him out in 1954, and he received a cheque for the deal. While he didn't wave the cheque around or even show it to us—that was not his style at all—he said that he had never seen a single cheque for such a large amount.

Many years later, I had another connection with the ESB. Out of the blue, I received a letter from one of its employees, Gareth Davis. He apologised for writing, given that I did not know him, but he had been doing MBA coursework at a college in Philadelphia and Merck's donation of ivermectin was one of the business case-studies. Because of my involvement with ivermectin, Davis learned I had a connection with Donegal. He was from Donegal too—he grew up on a farm between Ramelton and Letterkenny—and he recalled the Campbell lorry coming to collect the potatoes from the farmers throughout the region. He, along with others, advocated for me to receive an honorary degree from Trinity College Dublin in 2012, well before the Nobel prize, and that meant a lot to me. I now have half a dozen honorary degrees, and I am grateful for each, but there is something particularly special about one from your *alma mater*.

Back in 1930s Ramelton, there was another innovation that was in place in the house to improve efficiency, but it did lead to some unusual behavior. It was a small button on the floor at the place where my mother sat at the dinner table. If she pressed on this button with her foot, she could summon the maid. My father was particularly fond of potatoes, and he grew several varieties, so we always had whatever was in season at the time. The dinner table would feature a large bowl of hot potatoes, perfectly boiled and dried so the skin was starting to crack open. My father was attentive to visitors, and a guest might be halfway through a potato when my father would decide that the supply on the table was getting cold. My mother would then press the button, and the maid would come in with a bowl of fresh, hot potatoes. Guests, I think, were bemused by this compulsion to serve potatoes piping hot.

My father and mother both were workers by nature, but in accordance with religious scripture they did not work on Sundays. That must have been hard for my father, but he took it seriously. The injunction against work did not apply to 'errands of necessity and errands of mercy', and occasionally that called for difficult judgement. Farming was a major part of his business, and when prolonged bad weather threatened the gathering-in of the crops, my father was one of those farmers who did not yield to the temptation to order the harvesting crew into the fields. He always stuck it out until the weather improved.

Thus, Sundays were sacrosanct, and the joy for us as kids was that it was when we had Daddy to ourselves. I eagerly looked forward to those days, when as a family we might drive off on an outing to the beach (Donegal weather permitting) and back home in the evening, where Daddy—that was what I called him—would sit in his big upholstered leather chair near the fire and we would begin our favourite Sunday ritual. My parents subscribed to *The Christian Herald*, a magazine-style newspaper that arrived weekly. On those Sunday evenings, Daddy would sit each of my brothers on a knee and I would rush to sit on the floor between his feet—my baby sister being too young to participate. He would show us the pictures (never in colour in those days) in the paper.

We loved the human-interest stories, with their images of people and places in other parts of the world. Daddy would explain to us that this or that event was in another country and what the city was, or what these people were doing. Whatever was happening, it could hardly have been 'new' news by the time it got to Ramelton. This, after all would have been about 1934–35. But we were riveted! There were puzzles for children to do, and I remember doing one and sending it away as part of a competition. There was the agony of waiting for a response— and then it arrived: I had won an award! I have long since forgotten what the award was, but almost a lifetime later I still recall the thrill of a package arriving addressed to me by name. There was a special excitement in the rarity and importance of such an event.

On those Sundays my mother still needed to carry out some domestic duties. The maid had the afternoon and evening off. My parents had traditional roles: he ran the business to generate income and she looked after the house and family, including the extended family of workers in the shop. My mother was always busy. She had maids, at least one if not two at some points, but I think she worked even harder than they did. Our tutor, Elizabeth Martin, lived with us for decades. She was responsible for taking us out for afternoon walks and undoubtedly provided some child-care beyond school-room hours—but she was by no means a nanny. Indeed, her constant presence meant constant informal teaching, as befitted her role as tutor. It is remarkable, and wonderful, that she and my mother apparently lived in perfect harmony.

My mother made the best wheaten bread imaginable. When my brother Lexie was living in England as an adult, he used to try and get comparable wheaten bread in local shops, but nothing was ever as good as the bread our mother baked. She was also famous locally for her sponge-cakes. If anyone was coming to tea she would say she had to make a 'wee sponge'—it wasn't so wee, with its double layers and a fancy cream filling. I didn't happen to like sponge-cakes (I thought them big and boring) and, anyway, 'afternoon-tea' was for grown-ups. If my mother had a reputation for her sponge-cakes, I am prepared to concede that they were good.

We had lots of cream growing up. It came from our cows and went on cornflakes, stewed plums and of course into the sponges. Quite often we had rennet for dessert. For those unfamiliar with it, rennet is a kind of gelatinous curd, sweetened with enzymes of bovine origin. It was often combined with fruit. It may not sound appetising, but we loved it. Kids seem to love the food they grow up with, and, looking back, I remember enjoying the food tremendously.

My mother was an eager person, and, as far as I could tell, she saw her domestic duties as the natural lot of women at that time. It was her mission to feed and look after us. She seemed to thrive on it, and took pride in it. I do not recall my mother ever saying a bad word about anyone. I am biased, of course, but I am endlessly grateful for her patient and steadfast love. After her death in 1985, my brother Lexie referred to her saintly character, and none of us would disagree with that.

In my father, my mother made what I am sure she and the neighbours all considered a good catch; this up-and-coming young businessman. It must have been evident, too, that my father had been incredibly fortunate in marrying the lovely Sadie Patterson, a woman so capable, so amiable, so devoted to her family and so committed to her role in life.

So far as I know, they were happy. Certainly they were not the jovial, back-slapping type. They were focused, dedicated to their roles in life and, above all, busy—yet never harassed by busyness. I think they lived good lives.

Around town my father was known as R.J., but when we were growing up, my mother typically referred to 'Himself' or 'The Boss', just as the workpeople around did without thinking about it. When she would talk to the men coming in from the shop to have their morning tea, if she wondered where my father was she would say 'Have you seen the Boss this morning?' For his part, my father would refer to my mother as 'Herself' or 'The Missus'.

I never heard my parents address each other by their first names, nor by any endearment such as 'Dear' or 'Darling'. Later in life when my brother Lexie went to live in England, he and his wife called each other 'Darling' all the time. We certainly noticed that when they came back to visit Ramelton! Looking back, I am tremendously impressed by the fact that I never heard my mother call my father Robert or John or Bob, nor my father call her Sadie or Sarah Jane. I wonder how they addressed each other in their private hours and I know little about their discussions at all: did they talk about what furniture to get, did they have differences of opinion, did they discuss finances? I just don't know.

They were a team and they had four children: Robert, Alexander, myself and Marion in that order. Of my siblings, the one with whom I had the most common interests was Alexander, though I never called him that. As a child he was Lexie to every-one, and he continued to be called by that name among family.

But he declared himself Alex as an adult, which was probably a smart move. Lexie and I both went to study at college after school while Bert, by virtue of priority in birth order, was destined to stay close to home and inherit the family business. As it happened (or was it due to some subtle family influence of which we were unaware?) Bert had little interest in school or scholarship, and from an early age was eager to abandon homework in the school-room at home and to hang about in the shop and the 'stores' in the back, interacting with the employees.

Lexie and I would linger in the school-room after school and fiddle with this and that—books, boxing-gloves, darts and such. Kids always wore short trousers in those days, and one time, one of my darts bounced off the target and became embedded in Lexie's thigh. The dart may have been quickly pulled out, but being heavily weighted, and being in very soft tissue, it may simply have fallen out. The incident elicited neither a cry of pain nor an outburst of rage. Instead, we were fascinated to watch the dark blood ooze gently from the wound. Indeed, I suspect that it was the blueness of the blood that imprinted the scene in my memory. It was such a clear-cut freak accident that we would not even have thought about such things as blame or guilt.

Lexie, a year-and-a-half older than me, was always bossing me around, which might be perceived—at least by others!— as an older brother's privilege. He was always arguing, and he out-argued me at every turn. His behaviour did nothing for my self-esteem, but it must have served him well on both counts (bossing and arguing) when he was called to the bar as a very young man and went on to become an executive in a big international business company, IBM.

Among us kids, he was the raconteur and the wit, the life and soul of the party, and he looked out for me when we were at school at Campbell College and later when we were both students at Trinity College Dublin. In later years I was to visit him in London, Brussels and Paris as well as various places in England and Ireland. When I visited him in London, probably about 1951, he introduced me to the experience of dining at a Chinese restaurant. In hindsight, I realise that he was both instructing me and trying to impress me with his *savoir faire* as a sophisticated young man-about-town. In the latter objective, he was very successful.

It always amazes me how quickly Lexie adapted to new environments, whether it was learning to play rugby at the boarding school we attended (which he did effortlessly, despite no previous experience of it), then studying law and being called to the bar even though he did not intend to practise as a barrister, and later on getting to grips with the technical knowledge he needed at IBM. He succeeded wherever he went. Lexie settled in England, married Betty Parker, and they had four children: Sarah, Clare, Nicola and Peter.

Robert, or Bert, was three years my senior, and, when we were children, this felt like a different age-bracket entirely. As an adult, Bert inherited the business and became a respected and popular figure in the town of Ramelton. Among his interests, apart from R.J. Campbell (Donegal) Ltd., was the founding and nurturing of a tennis club, and eventually the installation of modern tennis courts just a stone's throw from the court on his home property. Bert remained for me the anchor to Ramelton, as well as being a focal point of the family in its Irish context. On all my return visits to Ireland, Bert was there in Ramelton—there when my parents were both alive, there when my mother was a widow, and there when she was gone. He was there until the end. He married Anne Mills of Derry and they had three children: John, Grier and Ruth.

My sister Marion arrived in our family four years after I was born. I think it was tough for her when we were growing up. In theory, it could have turned out that we three boys pampered this lovely little sister, but that's not how it was. We three boys were a gang unto ourselves, and I'm afraid that we were much preoccupied in the rough-and-tumble of boyhood life. Marion had a few years as the only child left at home with my parents before she, too, went off to boarding school. As a teen, she developed an interest in horses and she went to England to hone her riding skills and 'muck out' the stables of a renowned horse trainer. Tragically, not long after, the trainer was aboard a de Havilland Comet plane that crashed—this was in the early days of commercial jet liners—and he lost his life.

22

Marion was living at home in Ramelton in the summer of 1954 when I was also there—that being the interim period between the two phases of my graduate studies in Wisconsin. It was a delightful time of getting to know each other as young adults rather than as children. The weather was perfect—at least in my memory—and we drove to all our old seaside haunts for picnics and swimming. She went to work in London, and later married Albert Rossley of Dublin. They moved to Donegal and, for a while, Albert worked in the shop in Ramelton with Bert. He then set up a successful wine distributorship. Marion and Albert had three children: Stephen, Nickolas and Jane. Sadly, Albert died quite young. As I write, Marion is my only living sibling and we remain happily, though infrequently, in touch.

Long after it was too late, we learned that my father had, at some level, cherished a vision of his three sons heading branches of the company in three Donegal towns. But that did not happen. Instead, we three brothers eventually settled in three different countries, married and raised families in those countries, and enjoyed periodic visits and exchanges and interactions for the rest of our lives. On one occasion, Bert, Lexie and I were in Ramelton at the same time with our young families. There we were, three couples who spoke in different ways: Mary was American and I had acquired something of an American accent; Bert and his Derry-born wife Anne had a northern Irish accent; Lexie's wife, Betty, was English and Lexie had acquired a British accent. Our kids were amused by the thought that these three by now quite different men were brothers and had grown up in the house in which we were then gathered.

My father died in 1956, in his 70s. In broad terms, my mother spent a third of her life a maiden, a third married and a third a widow. She was in her 80s when she died, in 1985. Only my sister and my brother Bert lived to hear my Nobel prize news in 2015, and indeed Bert and his wife Anne attended the ceremonial festivities in Stockholm. Marion was suffering from bronchitis at the time and so could not travel. Lexie had died five years earlier, so neither he nor my parents could be there—to my profound regret and sadness.

Family reserve

Ours had been a very undemonstrative family in our youth, which is a pity. It was a matter of time and place: parents didn't tell their children that they loved them, or that they were proud of them. Hugs and proclamations of praise were alien to the day-to-day activities of our Ramelton family.

Although they were probably not the only times it happened, I remember twice my father complimenting me, and the fact that I remember those occasions tells you something. The first instance was on one of the Sunday evenings with family. My brothers had left home by then, but we still had prayers and readings from the Bible. On one occasion, my father asked me to pick and read something and I did. He said 'That was well chosen and well read.'

The second compliment was when I graduated from Trinity College Dublin with first-class honours. My father said I had taken it up well and he hoped I would lay it down well. That is very indicative of who he was. He was basically saying that I had made a good start in life, and that I should live so as to ensure that my life would still be considered worthwhile when I reached the end of it. Not effusive, yet inspiring to me.

Nowadays we openly tell our kids that we love them and how proud we are of them. Maybe things have gone to the other extreme, but on balance the modern openness is much better than the reserve that was predominant in my upbringing.

At home at school

Upstairs in the attic that my father had converted into a classroom was where our early formal education took place, thanks to our live-in tutor Miss Martin. The walls were papered and there was a painted blackboard, a step up from the little slates my father and his fellow students had used in their one-room school in Drumfad. There was a wonderful geographical globe in our classroom, and tables arranged into a semicircle, and this was where Miss Martin instilled in me the love of learning.

Originally from Rostrevor in Northern Ireland, she was a graduate of Trinity College Dublin and a qualified teacher. How she came to be our tutor remains a mystery to me, but my father was big on education. He had received relatively little schooling in his youth and he was determined that his children would have better opportunity. It was highly unusual to be 'home-schooled' in Ramelton at that time, and Miss Martin's students were probably unique in that regard. There were not many of us: myself and my siblings, and later, when I went to boarding school, my sister was joined in school at home by the children of our aforementioned minister, Reverend Scott.

Miss Martin was a wonderful person, and she became very much part of our family life. When the war ended and petrol (and cars) became available again, my father bought a second car. My mother (like many of her generation) had steadfastly refused to learn to drive, so it was Miss Martin who made the journey to Sligo (about 75 miles or 120 km away) to collect the new car. It was a shiny Ford v8, very big, very American, with power steering and a radio! It just glided along, and Miss Martin loved driving it. Needless to say, it was the only one of its kind in Ramelton at the time! Our old Riley car had been 'on blocks' during the war, but my father had it re-commissioned, and both cars remained in use for some years.

But back to the attic. It was here that Miss Martin elicited in me a positive motivation to learn. The idea was not to learn something so you could show off that you knew it. Rather it was about the internal satisfaction of knowing something that you had not known until that very moment!

Miss Martin revelled in teaching English and Latin, and I revelled in learning those subjects. We learned reams of poetry by heart. On certain evenings she listened to a BBC broadcast called 'The Brains Trust', on which a panel of experts tried to answer questions sent in from the audience. It was a popular show and it could receive thousands of letters each week. One of the panelists, C.E.M. Joad, would spontaneously recite a burst of poetry if the occasion called for it. Miss Martin would tell me about it the next day, and she would say that someday—someday far off in the future—I might be able to recall the very poem that I was now trying to memorise. And that worked! Throughout my life I have been able to recite many lines and verses that I learned in that attic. (They are gradually fading.) My father was also fond of reciting portions of the poems he had learned when he was in school. But my chief exposure to poetry was in the context of reading and memorising, rather than writing. Nothing was ever mentioned about the creation of poetry, or even about a wish to create it.

Nevertheless, very early in life, during this period of learning in the attic, I did compose a poem. It was written on a loose sheet of paper and was borne of frustration and introspection. The refrain was 'I have lost my pencil somewhere and I don't remember where'. Undoubtedly this particular effort occurred at the time when I was the only pupil in our attic room; my brothers had gone to boarding school, my sister Marion was too young for school, and I was spending a lot of out-of-school time by myself. The poem was to surface again a good many years later. I remember sitting in the living room at home with other family members—probably when my brothers and I were home on vacation from Campbell College. Miss Martin, who was still living in our house and teaching my sister, came into the room with a piece of paper in her hand, saying 'Look what I found!'

She started reading my poem with evident glee, and I think it was the glee aspect of the situation that elicited a strong reaction from me. I jumped to my feet, grabbed the paper out of Miss Martin's hand, and threw it into the fire that was always burning in the living-room fireplace. Miss Martin gave a little laugh of astonishment at what must have seemed an excessive reaction on my part. Nothing more was said. In retrospect, I am sure she was embarrassed because she did not realise that I had been stung to action by an instantaneous perception that she was making fun of me and my poem. My action was not a matter of deliberation. The poem was entirely matter-of-fact and contained nothing that would merit being kept a secret; nevertheless, I had reacted to what I perceived to be an intrusion into something very personal.

This vignette aside, my abiding memories of our 'home-schooling' with Miss Martin and her tiny group of students in our little attic classroom are of happy, productive days. I now suppose that there was something comforting about going downstairs to one's own family kitchen for a chocolate biscuit at mid-morning teatime. There was also some social cost to having a teacher all to myself for some of those years, rather than being in a busy classroom of children, but Miss Martin's gift to me was the desire to be an educated person and to develop a collegiality with others who really enjoy learning.

A brush with pneumonia

I was generally a healthy child, but when I was nine or ten I developed a serious bout of pneumonia. I must have been very ill, yet I can only deduce that from my memory of the activity and attention that surrounded me. My illness prompted visits from the town doctor in Ramelton, Cornelius Boyle, who was the very epitome of the General Practitioner—the trusted and admired figure who handled all sorts of conditions in all sorts of people, men and women, young and old, rich and poor.

As the doctor deemed advisable (and perhaps, in rare cases, as requested), he would call in a consultant to provide a second opinion. When word got around that 'a Consultant has been called', neighbors would respond with a slow shake of the head that left no doubt that the case must be serious.

Thinking of this today, I wonder if Dr Boyle knew about the new medicine M & B 693 in 1939–40, when I almost died of pneumonia; or had the consultant put him on to it as the best bet for my survival? Either way I am profoundly indebted to Dr Boyle, in addition to the people responsible for the existence and availability of M & B 693.

Many years later, I recalled the episode in a poem, which was published in *Perspectives in Biology and Medicine*.

M & B 693

I nearly died at nine and a half
and when I think of it, which isn't
very often, certain details are always
there. I'm sure I was unconcerned
about my fate, and I suspect that
I remember the things I remember
because they made me feel important:

The family traffic in my room, the
extra bed in the corner for my
mother's night vigil, Miss Martin reading
the thermometer in the middle of the
night and feeling faint, Mr. Scott
praying for 'this Thy servant', Dr. Boyle's
little joke as he strode tweed-clad
into my room, my father silencing
his business machinery lest it
disturb my sleep.

But I suppose I remember
the screw-cap jar of spittle,
not because it was destined for
the big city where I had never been,
but because it was so wonderfully,
so gloriously, disgusting.

And I think I remember
the new medicine only because
it had a name I could not forget;
and decades later, when I had
a different interest in new medicines,
I looked up M & B 693 (now dull and
dignified sulfapyridine)
and tried without much success
to conjure up some sort of magic
from the printed page.

If the guys who made it and
tested it and sold it were typical
folk, they didn't do that stuff
for me or even for 'mankind.'
They would be embarrassed by thanks,
but to hell with it—
I thank them anyway.

Belfast,
Northern Ireland

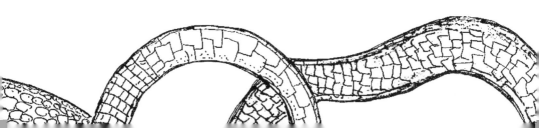

Campbell goes to Campbell College

When I was thirteen, I went to Campbell College, a boarding school near Belfast. Founded in 1894 with a bequest from Henry James Campbell, who had made his money in the linen trade, it was deemed to be one of the most prestigious schools in Northern Ireland. Perhaps its most famous student was the author C.S. Lewis, who had attended for a few months before a respiratory problem prompted his move to a health-resort town in England.

My brothers Bert and Lexie had both gone to Campbell College before me, leaving me on my own with our tutor Miss Martin in our attic schoolroom. For me, moving from such cloistered and attentive schooling to the hustle and bustle of a large boarding school was a culture shock, and I found it hard initially.

Some of my peers experienced homesickness, but I did not. It was my first time being 'properly' away from home. The only other time I had spent a night away from Ramelton had been a trip to Belfast for a dental appointment. But perhaps what spared me from the keen edge of homesickness at boarding school was that I wasn't that far from family: my brothers were still at the school. As they were older boys, I didn't talk to them or have anything to do with them. They were different beings entirely, and you didn't mix; but I knew they were there.

It was wartime when I started, and the school had been evacuated from the city of Belfast, which, as a major urban centre in Northern Ireland (and thus part of the United Kingdom), was a potential target for enemy bombs—and which was in fact damaged by enemy bombing during the war. Now the school was in operation at the sea-side town of Portrush in County Antrim. This meant that instead of dorms we were staying in hotel rooms, and I got on well with my room mates.

At school, I felt everyone was more sophisticated than I was. They seemed to know about things. Perhaps this was a social cost of my home-schooling. But I enjoyed the novelty of new experiences, which was probably the ideal mindset in which to enter this phase of my life and education. An experience I did not enjoy, however, was team sports. At a boarding school for boys, physical therapy and exercise is an important element of the set-up, but World War II was in full swing and this had taken its toll on the faculty in charge of sports and physical exercise. Many, if not all, of the masters and drill instructors who had been in charge of keeping us boys fit were now part of the war effort, and consequently older boys in the school took their place for physical therapy and sports sessions. This may well have been of some benefit to me. I recall those older boys teaching us to climb the sides of buildings with ropes, which felt both exhilarating and practical. They also taught us to vault over the gymnastic 'horse,' and that, too, was exciting. But when the regular instructor (a retired Regimental Sergeant Major) came back from the war, the enjoyment level dropped considerably. He kept us in the gym and had us play touch-football. I disliked that, because I was hopeless at contact sports.

To add injury to insult, I got my nose broken when playing, and the doctor at the school infirmary reset it there and then with vise-like pressure of his thumbs. This probably sealed my aversion to touch-football.

Aah, but the swimming pool! Our school building, having been a luxury hotel, had not just an indoor swimming pool, but a heated indoor swimming pool! With sea-water!! And a springboard and a diving platform!!! I practically lived at the pool. An elderly local man used to come to the school to conduct lifesaving classes under the aegis of the Royal Lifesaving Society. Naturally I signed up. And there were consequences. Apparently I learned enough lifesaving technique to earn the society's 'Silver Medallion' and proudly wore a big, showy Royal Lifesaving Society medallion patch on my swimming trunks on Donegal beaches, where I don't think anybody noticed. The instructor persuaded me to become an instructor (presumably at some junior level) and to give a series of classes to other boys at school—which he promptly organised and scheduled for certain afternoons. The Campbell College teachers (known as Masters) were naturally appalled to find their sports teams discomfited, without consultation, by an outsider. Those teachers, to their credit, did not vent their anger on me. I would have been about 14 years old at the time, and I suppose I was blithely following the lead of the instructor, taking for granted that everything was approved—I was finally showing a bit of initiative. And in sports, no less! The classes proceeded. I had totally forgotten about this episode until I was rummaging through an old box of mementos and came across my little Royal Lifesaving Society 'medal', made of inferior metal because of wartime restriction.

The lifesaving medallion was followed (some seven decades later!) by one that was by no means extracurricular or in any way extraneous to the school itself. In 2016 I was surprised and honoured to receive the Henry James Campbell Award—named in honour of the school's founder, and made tangible in the form of a handsome medallion.

Those events have reminded me of a long-forgotten oddity arising from the timing of my entry to the school in the academic year 1943–4. Because 1944 happened to be the fiftieth anniversary of its founding, the college set up a Golden Anniversary Scholarship; my cohort of students was automatically enrolled as competitors for it. At least one of the subject papers had been prepared by Chevy Chase (and I suspect the whole thing was his handiwork). The French exam-paper was replete with what C.P. Snow would have described as 'questions of baffling simplicity'. I was awarded a scholarship (as, perhaps, were others), and my school fees were reduced for my remaining years at Campbell. My parents must have been notified directly about that, and I was probably told about it at school. Conceivably I could finally have had 'something to write home about'. We were required to write home once a week. This was a challenge for most of us boys, and many parents must have grown tired of weekly bulletins containing little more that the results of the school's latest rugby match against a rival school. For my parents, such news must have had an interest level of about zero. There was no such letter-writing obligation or custom operating in the other direction, and none of us would have expected it.

As as result of the school's wartime relocation to Portrush, we no longer had access to our regular playing fields, so we used local farm fields for sports. I may have written home about the school team's performance at rugby football, but when it came to playing I was completely clueless. In rugby, seen from my perspective, you were told you were on this team and others were on that team, someone blew a whistle and there you were. I didn't even know that in rugby you only pass the ball backwards. Yet many other boys knew what to do because they had gone to a prep school, or at least to a school with more than two or three pupils. I later found more sporting outlet in tennis, which we had the opportunity to play in the final year or two at Campbell College. Tennis was a sport I could enjoy. Now, seven decades later, I am 'reduced' to playing table-tennis with friends. And I love it!

Part of my dislike of team sports in school came from not having been exposed to them in my younger years. The same could not have been said for my issue with Latin. The Latin motto of Campbell College is *Ne Obliviscaris* ('Lest ye forget'), and indeed that is seared into my memory. What is also seared, though, is how the move to boarding school dampened my previous liking for Latin. When I was being schooled at home, Latin was a joy. Miss Martin acquired an introductory textbook that was appealing in its splendid newness, and also in its being written in a style that seemed to speak directly to the young pupil—me! I was fascinated to discover on my own that 'doctor' comes to us via Latin *docere*, to teach; *doceo*, I teach; 'doctor' one who teaches. I treasured that snippet of knowledge and tucked it away to last a lifetime.

Within a few months after going to Campbell College, I detested Latin. More to the point, and of course central to the point, is that I detested Latin classes. The teacher bullied us boys. He would, for example, command a boy (I am fairly sure it was sometimes me) to stand on a chair in the middle of class and recite a verb-infinitive over and over until the pronunciation was judged acceptable. It would not have been so bad had it not been done in a spirit of overt humiliation.

In retrospect, I cannot attach a lot of weight to my narrowly focused, well-hidden rage, and there may be mitigating factors in regard to the charge I have levelled against the Latin teacher who angered me so. Until I reached the age of thirteen, Miss

Martin had been my only teacher. I would therefore have been ill-prepared to encounter the more robust teaching common in boarding schools. Added to that is the fact that Miss Martin was my father's employee. Thus, I would have been a beneficiary not only of her good nature but also of the hidden benefit deriving from the fact that she was employed by my father.

It is likely that my inexperience would have made me temperamentally or emotionally unable to accept a Latin teacher for whom bullying was, in my view, integral to his *modus operandi*. Nevertheless, my distress was still real and I cannot dismiss it entirely. I used to fantasise about slipping poison into the coffee that the Latin teacher would drink at breakfast in the dining hall. I like to think that that was just a kid's way of coping with resentment at having my Latin ruined! And yet I have never forgotten it. I have, as an adult, taken pains to 'play down' or even excuse my very negative thoughts about that Latin teacher. Now, since embarking on this memoir, and after writing those words, I have encountered two other Old Campbellians, of about the same vintage, who share the very same negative memories of that man. How important teachers are in our lives—the good ones and the not-so-good ones!

An awakening in science

When I was a child, I don't think anyone (including myself) would have suspected me of becoming a biologist. I had an intuitive interest about nature, and it held a certain fascination for me, but I had no idea then that one could study the natural world or apply any sort of systematic scrutiny to it. That's because at no time in my early formal education at home do I recall any mention of nature or science. Miss Martin taught us English, Latin, History, Euclid's geometry and such; there was no physics, chemistry or biology—not even versions that were travelling under assumed names!

So, when I went to Campbell College boarding school, it came as quite a shock to me that science existed and that I was to study it. Class time was a struggle. Physics and chemistry particularly mystified me. To this day, chemistry strikes me as almost magical, and I have huge respect for its practitioners.

Biology, though, was what saved my bacon. This was due in no small part to the biology master, Robert Wells, who took an inventive approach to engaging his students. He apportioned a section of forest in the locality for each of us to study. Then we would make independent visits to our plots and observe the ecological cycles, the waxing and waning of species and features over time. My scrutiny was directed at exposed tree roots, and I would watch as beetles and fungi feasted on the bounty that they found in my tiny patch of ground. This 'observational' type of project suited me well.

When my Nobel prize was in the news, my brother told a journalist that he recalled me dissecting worms in Ramelton. It is likely that Mr Wells had been teaching us about the earthworm *Lumbricus terrestris*, and that this had inspired me to do investigations on my own. I do recall, though, finding out about other types of worm—worms that would go on to have a profound influence on my life (and it might be said that my life would influence theirs!). On an outing from Campbell College we visited an agricultural fair, and I picked up a leaflet about liver fluke disease and its treatment. It was news to me that these creatures could live in the liver of a cow or sheep, and that drugs could reduce the parasite burden on livestock. While this leaflet didn't seem particularly salient at the time, looking back it was my first introduction to the world of helminthology, the study of parasitic worms, and to the drug treatments used against them. That must have burrowed somewhere into my brain, because the chemical treatment of helminthic infections went on to form an important part of my research career.

A plane obsession

Twenty-one pieces of luggage. That is what Princess Elizabeth had with her when she arrived in Belfast on a destroyer to launch the giant aircraft carrier *HMS Eagle* in March 1946. How do I know? I counted them!

I was in the Air Training Corps (ATC) of the Royal Air Force, and on this occasion we were being inspected by the princess—who at age nineteen was just a few years my senior and had not yet ascended the throne. I recall thinking how much more vibrant and radiant she looked in real life compared to her photographs—but my involvement in the whole process was quite minimal. Having little to do, I amused myself by taking a visual inventory of the luggage.

My fascination with aircraft of all kinds was a seam running through my youth, and it provided a variety of novel experiences (the first aeroplane flight taken by a member of my family), boredom (hence luggage counting), adventure (my first date!) and disappointment (missing out on going up in a bomber).

I went to RAF training events in Northern Ireland and in England, as well as at Campbell College in Belfast, but my interest in flying was sparked long before that. The first rush that I recall was, as I've mentioned, when I received the book *Biggles flies east* as a Christmas present from my cousins. I went on to read many of the Biggles books, becoming utterly 'transported' by the bravery, integrity and derring-do of that heroic pilot.

Then during World War II, when travelling from my hometown in the Republic of Ireland to Londonderry or Belfast in the United Kingdom, I would pass RAF airfields and see Spitfires and Hurricanes parked on the tarmac or climbing majestically skyward. How I longed to be old enough to fly those planes!

Caught up in the fearsome glamour of war, I desperately wanted to shoot down enemy planes and become an 'ace' fighter pilot. I wanted to stroll nonchalantly in my beribboned RAF uniform and cut a suave figure with the girls—never mind that I was at a boys' boarding school and hadn't a clue as to what I would say to a girl if I met one. So, taking part in RAF training camps was, for me anyway, a decision that today we might call 'a no-brainer'. We didn't learn to fly planes at these camps—nor did I ever learn—but they built enthusiasm for aircraft and gave us boys the experience of being at a military base and being a bit 'grown up'.

My interest in flying broadened my horizons in other ways too. Another boarder and ATC cadet at Campbell College suggested that we go to England over the Christmas holidays to an Air Force base near St Alban's. Well I jumped at the chance. I never would have thought of doing such a thing, but when the prospect was presented, I was not going to pass this one up!

This would be my first opportunity to ride in a biplane, a de Havilland 'Dominie', which was thrill enough itself, but there were also adventures on *terra firma*. I met a girl and we went on what was my first date. In Ireland I would not have said 'boo' to an actual live girl, but here, emboldened by the exoticness of travel and new environments, I got to know a girl while my schoolfriend and I were roller-skating at Cricklewood, and arranged to meet her the next day for a stroll at the zoo. It was fun, and naturally it was a fleeting relationship.

There was a price to pay for the English adventure, though. The time flying in the de Havilland meant my flight log was impressively full, and that meant I would later miss out on flying in a large bomber plane—for several hours! This was at a training camp in Northern Ireland. There was room for all cadets but one, and my relatively replete flight log dictated that, in fairness, I would stay on the ground. At the time, aged around fifteen and in the uniform of the Air Training Corps I sat, disconsolate, on the edge of the tarmac at Aldergrove airfield, and pondered my hard luck. Deep down, I knew that disappointment of such severity might be surpassed some far-off day in the future; but I suspected (rightly!), that the present moment would never be forgotten. Now, more than seven decades later, I find it hard to imagine an afternoon so utterly miserable as one spent in the windowless belly of an extremely noisy World War II bomber, going nowhere in particular!

Neither war nor training turned my interest in flight into a profession, but my curiosity about planes endured long into adulthood. Much later in life, when as a family we travelled to Australia so that I might take up a research post, the flight happened to coincide with our son Peter's sixth birthday and he was invited to the cockpit to meet the pilots. Naturally, I volunteered to be the parent who accompanied him!

The personal psychology of war

I recall the moment when war became personal to me. I had been just nine years old when World War II was declared in September 1939. Ireland, where I lived with my family, was neutral throughout the war, yet wartime psychology and politics still affected the country deeply. A few years later, I went to boarding school in Northern Ireland, which, as part of the United Kingdom, was officially involved in the global conflict. Thus, war was all around for much of my childhood and adolescence. Yet I know that, at that stage, my awareness of it must have been in some ways rather juvenile. War was simply there. It was a background scene that shaped what we did, where we were schooled, how we thought.

When something dramatic happened—for example my brother Lexie, as well as Bert, going away to boarding school even though Lexie was very young, maybe only eleven—we were told that it was 'because of the war'; further explanation was apparently considered unnecessary. But you went along with the pervasive public psyche of wartime, which is so different from that of peacetime. I was steeped in the talk and radio broadcasts of war. The trappings of war were everywhere in my boyhood; they were markers of everyday life—endlessly horrifying and endlessly fascinating. You got wrapped up in it, the blackouts, the slogans that declare 'hush-hush, walls have ears', 'loose lips sink ships'. I had learned to hate the enemy, and it is frightening how clear-cut that was. When I was ten, if a German had walked into our house in Donegal, I thought I would have tried to kill him, just like that. The change in attitude is almost immediate.

At Campbell College, in my teens, I enjoyed some training in infantry warfare using World War I Lee-Enfield 303-calibre rifles with bayonet, and I learned how to 'strip' a Bren machine gun. We had gas masks that we were meant to carry slung over our shoulders. When our school was based at Portrush, we had been enchanted by the arrival of American soldiers into our little seaside town. We never thought to ask why they were there. We would not have been told. They were on their way to join Allied comrades in secret, fateful and heroic exploits elsewhere.

My interest in planes was intensified. In the Air Training Corps, I learned to distinguish the silhouette of a Heinkel Bomber from that of a Junkers. Know your enemy! Had I been old enough, I would have been off to war with banners flying, joining up without hesitation.

But later, as a student in Trinity College Dublin, came a new and more adult, personal perspective. A few of us used to take a break from lectures to go to Bewley's Cafe in Grafton Street, just a few minutes away from Trinity by foot, to have a coffee and a chocolate biscuit—a mid-morning tradition reminiscent of my time being taught in the attic by Miss Martin. We were there having a nice coffee one morning in June 1950, around the time of my twentieth birthday, when we heard the news about the start of the Korean War. It was a tense time in global relations and a pivotal moment for the newly formed United Nations, one of its first really big tests. In the days leading up to the announcement, there had been a question: would any of the western nations respond to this invasion from the north to the south of Korea? It was a watershed moment, and there had been much discussion about it. We were aware of the significance.

So, when the news arrived that Britain was joining the Korean War, it suddenly occurred to me as I sat with my friends in Bewley's that conceivably I could be drafted. Having been born in Londonderry, I had UK citizenship and I had a British passport as well as an Irish one. I also had a Northern Ireland driving licence as well as my licence for the Republic of Ireland. Did this mean I could be drafted, if there was to be such a campaign? I had a sudden and sharp feeling of being at a whole new level of 'grown up'. The world was shifting, things were changing, and I could be part of it. The prospect of going off to war wasn't particularly frightening—but it would be an interruption. It would disrupt my plan for further education. In the end, I didn't get the call to join the RAF, so I could continue my studies, but I see this as a moment when I developed a new sense of global awareness.

These days, when I speak to contemporaries who were alive in World War II, we are concerned about the fact that when this generation is entirely gone, no-one will personally recall the mood of the time and no-one will talk to the young people about how the public psyche is altered in wartime. This is scary, because that change happens quickly and when it does, everything changes.

Dublin,
Ireland

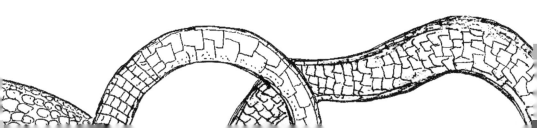

Learning from Trinity

Timing is important. When I was living in the United States and working at Merck, our community in New Jersey went through a 'craze' of doing aptitude tests. There was a programme of testing in New York City, and out of curiosity and a sense of fun, I took the test. It examined your vocabulary, physical dexterity, visual, aural and musical acuity and so on. My results were a little surprising to me. The final report said that I should avoid the sciences and work with people! Me, a scientist working on parasitic worms! Was I in the wrong career? I decided that the test results may have been skewed by the focus of my early education on English literature rather than science, and I was not tempted to change my career just yet.

Had I taken that aptitude test when I was about to leave school, and had I been guided by the results, my life path might have been quite different. In the 1940s, when I was preparing to leave Campbell College, the headmaster, Ronald Groves, wanted me to go into medicine, but my biology teacher, the previously mentioned Robert Wells, wanted me to go into biology. I don't know why, but I decided to take the headmaster's advice and I put down medicine on my application to attend Trinity College Dublin. In this case, it was the passage of time that nudged my career compass. During the summer before I went to Trinity, I changed my mind about medicine, and, when I got to Dublin, I registered to study natural sciences instead. Two decades later I wrote to Mr Wells to say that I was glad that I had opted as he had advised. He reported that biology at Campbell College was 'flourishing'. He had 23 students taking the subject, whereas in my day the number had been 4 or 5.

The day before I went to Trinity I went out for a cycle on my bike in Ramelton, and I thought about how my life would be different tomorrow. I was more excited and eager than apprehensive, but I had the advantage (probably unacknowledged by me!) of knowing that my older brother Lexie was already a student at Trinity. He became my solicitous advisor. I do not suggest for a moment that Lexie and I shared our social lives at Trinity, it was rather a matter of my receiving occasional visits to straighten me out on matters of campus protocol. But it was always a matter of treating me as a grown-up (if naïve) friend. I am sure that I would have been deferential and grateful in this new relationship—in the proper unspoken way. In retrospect, it seems a remarkable transformation; it was to evolve into a more balanced bond of fraternal ... well, I might as well say it ... love.

One of the most significant things Lexie did for me at Trinity was to alert me to the fact that an engineering student named Jeffrey Sockett from Sligo was in need of a student to share his 'rooms' (a small, two-bedroom apartment). I met with Jeffrey, and at once moved into his rooms on the ground floor in the old 'Botany Bay' part of the college campus. As a result, I was able to spend virtually my whole four year of college living on campus, ending up with a very desirable two-room apartment in the Graduates Memorial Building. This was a rare and extremely beneficial opportunity—as distinct from living in a rented room in the suburbs of Dublin as I had done for the first week or two. Living in the suburbs would have severely hampered participation in college life.

College life featured, among other things, dining 'on Commons'. That in turn meant listening to a long grace, spoken in Latin by a Scholar of the House; drinking free beer with dinner (a somewhat unpopular beer, bestowed on the college as a legacy and not interchangeable with other kinds of beer—which was OK with me since it was the only beer I had ever tasted and I loved it); and sitting in the magnificent Dining Hall, surrounded by ancient paintings of equally ancient academics and divines. The background sound to all of this was the chatter of a multitude of undergraduate students—most of whom seemed to me to be very intellectual in a sophisticated kind of way. I drank in the pearls of contemporary wisdom and the traditional ambiance as eagerly as I quaffed the free beer. Thus Lexie, by telling me about Jeffrey Sockett's need of a room-mate, had a big impact on my life at Trinity College Dublin.

There were two 'central' student societies at Trinity, 'the Phil' and 'the Hist'. Each had a choice location in the midst of things, a well-stocked reading room, and a strong tradition of evening debates. For no particular reason, I chose to join the Dublin University Philosophical Society over the Dublin University Historical Society. I remember the debates because such formal argument and parliamentary procedure were new to me. Speeches (even the briefest of remarks) were addressed only to the Chair of the society. Nevertheless, the debates, even those on serious subjects, were a form of entertainment—an alternative to going to the theatre or the movies. That, I believe, is an aspect of education that deserves much more attention than it customarily receives. It is quite distinct from the tradition of debate as a subject of academic coursework.

My friends at Trinity included Ronnie Hendly, Robin Maude, Lawrence Threadgold and Harvey Evans. I particularly valued my friendship with Ronnie Hendly. We didn't have a lot in common, yet we seemed to fall naturally into a comfortable relationship in which we could enjoy spending time in each other's company without feeling any need to talk. Ronnie was dating the lovely and vivacious Helen Kyle, whom he later married. He was under no pressure to prepare for a career, knowing that he would inherit his father's confectionery business in Omagh. He did exactly that, but tragically died of natural causes at an early age.

Of course there was the academic side of things at Trinity too. I soon fell into daily student life, studying in a manner that appealed to me. The lecturing style and the positioning of exams at the end of a vacation period (not the end of term) meant that there was a great incentive to study on your own. Thanks to my early experience of relatively solitary schooling, this suited me well. Some subjects were challenging. The standard grade for passing was 40% and one year my final mark in chemistry, which was still a subject of mystery to me, was 39.7%. Fortunately, they rounded it up the to the nearest whole number and I scraped through. Also, as had been the case in school, physics was a challenge for me, even with the benefit of a Nobel laureate in the subject teaching us at Trinity, Ernest T.S. Walton. No fault lay at his feet, though, for my difficulty in grappling with these 'hard sciences'.

Where I shone was still biology. I would go to the lectures and then write out my understanding of the information and physically draw the structures such as skeletons that we needed to memorise, filling the pages of numerous penny copy books from R.J. Campbell's. One of our lecturers, J.D. Smyth, encouraged us to spend time in the museum at Trinity and examine the skeleton specimens. I did, and it paid off. In our final exams we had a big 'practical' exam and I was able to identify the lower jaw of a Tasmanian devil (which I have not been called upon to do since then), because I had scrutinised that very jaw on my visits to the museum. Even though the teeth weren't in that jaw any more, I could have described its dentition in detail. I had learned, in the traditional way and mostly in solitude, a large amount of incredibly detailed stuff that nobody in their right mind was likely to find useful. As for the really useful stuff, the physiology and the biochemistry, we had relatively little instruction. But the big thing for me at Trinity was that I learned the skill and art of learning. I enjoyed independent study, reconstructing something I had read so that I could write about it. I tested myself constantly. The required essays that I wrote had serious content, and I recall Professor Smyth doing something he said he had never done before: he singled out one of my essays for reading to the class. Coming from a family where the compliments were countable on the fingers of one hand, that was a big deal.

Students doing an honours course in the natural sciences at Trinity did not take courses in any subject outside of the sciences. It was assumed that one came to college with a solid grounding in the humanities, and that assumption in that environment would have been generally valid. Just to be on the safe side, every student was required to pass the dreaded 'Littlego' exam within the first two years of college. This demanded a basic competency in various subjects, including English, Mathematics, Latin, and Logic. The Latin exam was a *viva*—oral rather than written. You entered a small room where a professor was sitting at a desk. He (it was a 'he' at that time) handed you a book of classic writings of Ancient Rome, pointed randomly to page and asked you to translate. As I recall, the process did not go on for very long because one's knowledge of Latin, and especially one's lack of it, was soon exposed. Some prospective medical students (including a friend of mine) chose to go to a different university simply because of Trinity's Latin requirement. There is some irony in that, for medicine is a profession in which Latin can be very helpful in mastering its terminology.

For most of us in the honours programme, Logic was an unknown quantity and was just an obstacle that had to be overcome. The usual approach was to study Abbott's *Elements of Logic* on our own and learn enough to pass the exam. The book was published 1883, but I had (and still have!) a battered 1900 edition. Poring over the book, I found that Logic was not merely an obstacle but also a fascinating novelty. Its message was so enlightening that I have, ever since, advocated the teaching of Logic, or at least some of its basic concepts, in secondary schools.

My primary subject at Trinity College was zoology and my secondary subject was botany. The head of botany was David Allardice Webb. Modern students of botany in Ireland will no doubt be familiar with the *Irish flora* that bears his name. One year, Professor Webb led a group of third- and fourth-year students of the subject, including myself, on an excursion to the south-western corner of Ireland. The objective was to study plant life in the vicinity of Caragh Lake, County Kerry. My chief memory of the excursion is not, strictly speaking, botanical. While hiking up the lower slope of a mountain, we came to a spring or pond in which a rare aquatic plant was known to grow under the surface of the water. Professor Webb pointed it out to us, but he wanted also to obtain a part of the plant for preservation in the Botany Department. To do that, someone would have to get completely into the icy water. When Professor Webb called for volunteers, I stepped forward together with another student, John Scanlon. Webb announced the plan, telling the rest of the group to continue hiking and reminding them of the story of Lot's wife, who tragically did look back when told not to. John and I stripped off and got the plant specimen. However, I do not recall that anybody was particularly impressed by our little bit of bravado.

50

One of my friends at Trinity, an Englishman and engineering student called David Finch, was a diehard socialist. This fascinated me—not the socialism itself but his immersion in, and his devotion to, the cause. He had a subscription to *Hansard*, which provides a printed record of debates in the British parliament, and he was ready at any moment on any day to give the Labour point of view on any subject. I really envied him. I wondered how he was able to do that, to read a paper and know the arguments of today on today's problem, then to talk about it with such conviction even without reading the opposing opinions on the matter. I thought it would be such a nice thing to be able to do, I was bewildered by it and in awe of him. David told me it was a simple matter of faith. I had never thought of that until then—about having a political faith—and I realise now that throughout my life I have never developed such a thing. As a scientist it is good to be unsure, to have doubts; and I have always been good at doubting, so maybe that partly explains why I have had no passionate adherence to a political party.

We also didn't talk about politics at home. Such matters were simply not part of family life. In an Irish context there are various reasons for that, not least that the people in general were shell-shocked from the turbulence of the War of Independence in 1919—21, when Ireland sought to overthrow British rule, and the bitter hostility of the ensuing Civil War of 1922–23, which had torn families and friendships apart. There were occasional passing references but no education about the context. My father would point out the blackened ruin of a building that had been 'blown up during the troubles', but there was no explanation or discussion of the politics that had led to such violence. As an aside, those 'troubles' my father spoke of had their own descendants in the form of civil unrest and violence in Northern Ireland in the latter decades of the twentieth century. I lived in the US by then, but my brother Bert teamed up with a Catholic neighbour in Ramelton and raised money to house refugees who needed to leave Belfast or Londonderry.

But back in the 1940s, when I was at Trinity, politics was a curiosity rather than a conviction. I did have a rare opportunity to actually see Éamon de Valera, who had been one of the 1916 revolutionary leaders and who had gone on to become taoiseach (prime minister) of Ireland, and eventually the president of the country. Mr de Valera had been invited to Trinity for a debate of 'the Phil'. When I saw him, he was in the Reading Room, talking to the officers of the society. He was white-haired by then, and in his evening suit he looked every inch the elder statesman. I recall being intensely curious about this historical figure, still alive and looking very much at home among the scholars.

As a student, my curiosity was also piqued by word of a gathering near O'Connell Bridge just a few minutes' walk from Trinity. It was 1949 and Ireland was establishing itself as a republic, withdrawing the External Relations Act that kept it part of the British Commonwealth, and replacing it with the Republic of Ireland Act. I thought this was an important historic event and I should go and join the crowd. When I got there, it was an orderly, calm crowd. A van from the news media was there with cameras mounted on its roof and people on the van were telling the crowd to yell and wave but getting very little reaction. Perhaps, like myself, other members of the crowd were also motivated more by curiosity to be there than anything else.

When I moved to the USA I went through the common arc of becoming a bit more liberal, then, as I got older, becoming a bit more conservative. I was politically engaged to the extent of writing, on occasion, letters of protest or endorsement to US senators and the president. But as for political faith? I'm still waiting to see if that develops.

Making memories

When school students are thinking about going to college, they (and their parents) often think about the subjects they will study and the academic credentials of a particular institution. That is important, certainly, yet so much of the growth we experience in college is due to being there, making friends and having adventures and new experiences. These are the things of which memories are made.

In Trinity College I shared rooms with two good friends, Lawrence Threadgold and the previously mentioned Ronnie Hendly. In 1949 Ronnie and I got the travel bug—we went by sea to the coast of France and hitchhiked to Paris. Paris was another world, and very warm. Being from Donegal, and thus unaccustomed to an abundance of sunshine, I suffered from heat prostration. On one such occasion I was helped into a sidewalk café to recover, and for the very first time I witnessed the technological breakthrough that was television. It was 14 July and all eyes were on the black-and-white shadowy figures marching in celebration of Bastille Day. Charles De Gaulle was undoubtedly among the marchers, but my memory does not capture that detail.

In 1950 Ronnie and I toured the south of Ireland with Harvey Evans, in his car. The following year, the three of us and Lawrence Threadgold toured Norway, Sweden and Denmark in a car borrowed from Ronnie's brother. I was to encounter Lawrence again after graduation. He invited me to be best man at his wedding to Jenny Thompson in Northern Ireland, with the reception held at the Crawfordsburn Inn.

There was at the time a fairly well-established convention regarding the duties of a best man, especially in regard to speech-making. It was understood that the best man would propose a toast to the bridesmaids. In what would turn out to be something of a precedent, I took the job seriously and devoted considerable time to the preparation of my speech. It was, I suppose, the very beginning of a lifetime of making speeches on social as well as scientific occasions.

Years later, Lawrence and Jenny Threadgold came to visit my wife Mary and me at our 'summer retreat' on Cape Cod, Massachusetts. When 'on Cape', Mary and I enjoyed bicycling on its flat rails-to-trails bike-paths as well as other not-so-flat trails, and Lawrence and Jenny joined us. Little did we realise that this would lead to bicycle-tours together—in Vermont; the Dordogne Valley; the Maine coast; the Loire Valley; Cotswold villages; the hills of Tuscany; mountain bike-paths in Austria; to say nothing of a study-tour of cave paintings in Spain (Altamira) and a barge-and-bike week on the River Lot and French canals. Now, as I write, we and the Threadgolds remain friends, separated by an ocean but connected by shared experiences that are treasured in memory.

The ins and outs of dining out at Inns

It's amazing how much happens at the lunch table. Over the years I have sat and conversed at many lunch tables—with my family, with fellow students at Trinity and later at the University of Wisconsin-Madison, with colleagues at Merck and with other parasitologists at conferences. There was a moment I recall vividly when the lunch table was the location for one of my unusual moments as a student. At Trinity, a magazine called *TCD Miscellany* had printed my first published poem. This magazine had a few serious literary essays and maybe a short story, but the main thing that most of us actually read was a series of little snippets that were directed at students in college. We were intrigued about people that we knew, or the people we wished we knew in the year ahead of us.

These snippets were submissions written by students, they were poems or quotes from literature that worked in the name of another student, not the full name but a hint of it. It was all anonymous and a bit of fun. The poem I submitted was about my brother Lexie, who was studying law. As well as doing their degree in College, law students attended law sessions at the King's Inns (one of the 'inns of court'), and on certain occasions there were dinners. My brother, if you recall, was a big raconteur. He had a little too much to drink at one of these events at Inns and he caused a bit of a sensation.

I worked this into my poem for the magazine, including the lines:

> Will someone please dispel my doubts
> A pint for he who wins
> Has Campbell learned the ins and outs
> Of dining out at Inns?

Even though Lexie's name was disguised, the publication elicited a swift visit to me from him, telling me on no account to admit to anyone that I had written it. I agreed to anonymity.

It was tested one day, though, when I was having lunch in the common room with other students. There were big tables that seated lots of groups, and at the other end of my table sat a well-known figure from around campus. He was 'artsy' and he had a straggly beard. I heard him talking to the guy he was having lunch with, asking him had he seen this poem that had the line 'Has Campbell learned the ins and outs of dining out at Inns'? Well, I was bursting to jump up and tell him that I had written that, and here I was at the same table.

I managed to contain it and keep my silence, but that admiring nod, all the more treasured because he could not have known the author was within earshot, gave me a jolt of immodest pride.

Respect for the parasites

I have a liking for worms, even though I have spent half my life trying to kill them. I don't mean the earthworms in the soil of our fields and gardens; we definitely don't want to kill those. I mean the parasitic worms that in some way cause diseases in their hosts. From the flattened flukes in sheep livers to the coiled *Trichinella* roundworm larvae in pig muscles to the ribbon-like tapeworms in human intestines, I find them utterly fascinating and, in many ways, beautiful.

As mentioned, I first became aware of parasitic worms at an agricultural show that I attended with my school. The only thing I really remember about that show was coming back with a leaflet from the chemical company ICI about liver fluke in sheep and cattle. This was when I realised that there were worms living in animals, that these worms could cause disease and that there were drugs to cure them. But that awareness alone did not change my life. I did not immediately decide to devote a life of study to them.

The moment of enlightenment about parasites, or perhaps it was more of a slow dawning, happened later, when I was studying natural sciences at Trinity . The junior of the two professors in the zoology department was a parasitologist called James Desmond (J.D.) Smyth. He and I just hit it off; he would stop and talk to me in the corridor about his work and I showed an interest.

I had been a pretty shy student in Trinity, and when we were choosing our final-year projects I knew that two other, more confident and experienced students had applied to work with Professor Smyth. I figured that put me out of contention, which disappointed me greatly. But when the term started in our final year, I saw that the professor had selected me, as well as the other two, to study parasitology with him. That was a big moment for me. He was an astute mentor, he had confidence in me where I lacked it, and that changed my life. Everybody should be so lucky as to have a professor with whom you have a lasting and meaningful bond.

Professor Smyth would come in on Saturday mornings to give the three of us lectures, which seemed to me to be above and beyond the call of duty. From the outset, I loved learning about parasites, about their biological workings and how parasitic diseases affect humans and other animals around the world. From Trinity on, I looked innumerable times through microscopes at parasites, and experimented with them as I grew into a researcher.

That work brought me to the USA, Iran, Australia, Asia, Central and South America and the African continent, because parasites are widespread and remarkably successful. They inhabit animals and plants around the globe in a marvellous variety of shapes and sizes, using strategies that dodge the host well enough for the parasite to remain and survive. As humans, we may be conditioned to deplore their lifestyle, and we are definitely biased in favour of the host surviving, but deep down we must applaud their success.

We also have to remember that, as our understanding of the natural world deepens through scientific observation and study, it is becoming clear that no living thing exists in isolation. Parasites themselves are part of an ecosystem, just as we are. If you change something about an ecosystem, maybe seeking to remove a parasite, it could have unintended consequences on other living organisms in that ecosystem. So, it is imperative that our goal is the absence of parasitic disease rather than the absence of parasites.

Of course, some parasites and diseases are closely intertwined, and this creates difficulties. To illustrate that point, a person who attended a talk that I gave asked an unexpected and direct question about parasites and I have never forgotten it. It was whether, if I could pull a trigger and eliminate every last river-blindness-causing parasite in the world, I would do it or not. Would I? That really threw me. I finally replied that yes, I probably would, but I wouldn't feel good about it. It's an interesting thought experiment, and fortunately that is where it has remained, but the question gave me pause.

Madison,
Wisconsin

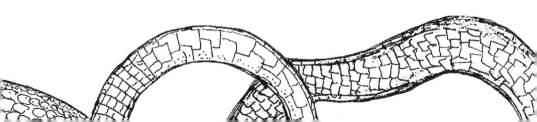

Moving to America

During the final year of my undergraduate studies at Trinity College Dublin, Professor Smyth called his three parasitology students together. He had received a letter from a fellow parasitologist, Arlie Todd at the University of Wisconsin-Madison, asking for recommendations for students to do PhD projects. J.D. Smyth recommended all three of us, and we were all accepted. The plan was to finish our undergraduate degrees in 1952 and head to America the following January.

I was extremely anxious ahead of my final exams. But they came and they went well, bringing me a first-class honours degree in zoology. As I mentioned, after I finished college, I spent several months working for my father, travelling around on the R.J. Campbell lorry, hauling sacks of potatoes as we collected them from farmers or delivered them to customers.

When the time came to leave Ireland for the USA, I first crossed the Irish Sea eastward by ferry to Liverpool. My brother Lexie was living in London at the time and he came to Liverpool to see me off properly. The next day, I boarded the liner *MV Britannic* bound for New York via Cobh and Bermuda. I did not have the company of my former classmates on that trip across the Atlantic though. Those other two who had also been selected to work with Professor Todd had both opted out of doing PhDs in Wisconsin, leaving me, the shy one, to go it alone. One of them had written a note saying 'For God's sake, don't panic when you get off the boat in New York City!' That was easier said than done.

New York City was something else. I was a boy who had grown up in a rural town in Donegal and had shrunk into shy diffidence when faced with the bustle of Dublin city. Now I was in New York, and the bustle was on an entirely different level, as was my diffidence! I wandered around soaking it in, eventually finding a 'delicatessen'. I was too overawed even to speak to the assistant, so I just pointed to what I wanted to eat. The experience would have been much worse but for the Committee on

Friendly Relations Among Foreign Students. Mrs Minucci from the committee met me on the dock at New York and soon had me installed in a nearby hostel. I was assigned a bed in a large dormitory room, and was advised to keep my belongings close about me.

There wasn't much to keep close about me. There were restrictions in those days on how much you could carry when you travelled from Ireland to the USA, so I had just $15 in my pocket when I stepped off the boat. Luckily my father had been contacted by a Donegal man by the name of James Callaghan who had moved to Chicago, Illinois and had become a successful lawyer. He had said he would loan me the princely sum of $100 to help when I got to the US. Mr Callaghan had heard from an old Donegal friend that I was on my way to Wisconsin, which goes to show that you should never underestimate the collective and up-to-date knowledge of the Irish diaspora. James Callaghan's kindness in offering that loan made the move to the USA easier in practical terms. I managed to repay him, in two installments.

On the boat over, I had decided that I would no longer be called by my middle name of Cecil, which had been my given name up to that point. I had grown to dislike the name Cecil, but had not wanted to disappoint my parents by switching to my first name of William. Now though, I felt independent enough to start afresh as Bill.

I thoroughly enjoyed the life of a researcher at the University of Wisconsin-Madison. I believe I was the only student there from Ireland, and at the start I was constantly aware of my different surroundings. I was aware for maybe a full year of the fact that the houses were made of wood rather than brick or stone, the street signs were different from the ones back home and the women dressed quite differently. There was always at least some sense of feeling alien, feeling temporary. I had initially assumed that one day I would return to work and live in Ireland or the United Kingdom, but over the years I realised that the USA was going to be my home. The sense of permanence became stronger in 1960, when I met Mary Mastin from New Jersey, who later became my wife.

How to have fun with flukes

Fasciola hepatica, or the liver fluke, is something of a poster boy in the world of parasites. This flattened, leaf-shaped little worm adorns textbooks and animal livers the world over. Liver fluke affects sheep, cattle and sometimes humans. The immature worm is bathed in the host's blood as it burrows through the unfortunate host's liver, causing much bleeding and damage to the liver cells and tissues along the way. Then the mature fluke crawls into the bile ducts where it finds a protective environment. Individual flukes may be small, but collectively the parasites can devastate the liver function of a large animal, and controlling these quivering flatworms is of enormous economic importance in agriculture.

Another type of liver fluke parasite infects deer, and has struck a different kind of deal with its host animal. If deer are infected with the large North American liver fluke, *Fascioloides magna*, they can tolerate its presence, and this relationship was the subject of my PhD research at the University of Wisconsin-Madison. The deal works like this: the deer keeps the adult parasites sequestered in expansions of the bile ducts that form capsules and connect to the deer's gut. In practice, this means the parasite is tucked away and therefore not wreaking havoc on the deer's internal organs, but the flukes can still release eggs into the deer's intestines and everyone is happy. Sheep and cattle also become infected with this giant fluke, but they cannot sequester the parasitic worms, which are thus free to continue to migrate through the liver, doing great harm.

When I arrived in Wisconsin and Professor Todd informed me I would be working on this giant fluke, the news was a little unexpected. An application to work in Professor Todd's lab had required the submission of a research proposal. Professor Smyth in Trinity had thought up a research objective for each of the three of us who were applying. We wrote them up as one-page essays, and added them to our documentation. I have no recollection of the specific details of my proposal, but it had been for a study on the effects of host nutrition on the growth of round-worm parasites. This was in an area of science known to be of interest to Professor Todd. So it was surprising on arrival at the University of Wisconsin-Madison to find that Todd had other ideas for me.

When I was assigned to work on the *Fascioloides magna*, however, I was far from being disappointed. Instead I was thrilled because of its similarity to *Fasciola hepatica*—its biological 'cousin' of greater fame and smaller dimension. As I knew something of the common liver fluke I was intrigued by this large relative, and we set out to examine how infections with this giant fluke differed between deer and sheep. This involved driving hundreds of miles to Northern Wisconsin in the departmental truck with another graduate student to buy the worst sheep that farmers could possibly find in their flocks. We wanted the ones that were grazing on marginal, swampy land and were effectively close to death. The farmers, of course, were delighted to get some money for these animals, and we were delighted to have them for our study of their infections. One man's trashed sheep is another man's treasure.

Those years in the 1950s of doing my Master's and PhD work in Wisconsin were a time of much professional growth for me, and a time of huge fun. I was initially a little overwhelmed by the amount of coursework that I was expected to take as a graduate student under the US system, but I soon found it was an opportunity to learn. The nature of my work, and the departments to which I was attached, also meant that I got to go to veterinary lectures and seminars as well as talks in zoology, which was much to my liking. Added to that, Professor Todd was a very good teacher. He left us free to follow our curiosity in the lab, to start in our own direction in research, and this brought with it a level of maturity and confidence in pursuing research.

How to drop a tray with grace

In the United States, almost everybody, at least on the male side, would seem to have had a 'paper route' when they were young, delivering newspapers as a way of making some money. That was not a tradition in the culture of County Donegal in my day. Loading potatoes onto the R.J. Campbell lorry could hardly be seen as a job. It did not earn money. It was a filial duty, and from this distance I can look back on it as having been a privilege. Serving as Demonstrator in zoology when I was a student at Trinity College Dublin brought in some money but was a form of reward, and definitely a privilege.

My first real job was as a dishwasher in what was disparagingly but aptly called a 'greasy spoon', a very lowly sort of restaurant. It was in Madison, and I was 23 or 24 years old. I was a graduate student and for the first time in my life I really needed hard cash. Into the tiny restaurant one night came Ed Thorpe, an undergraduate student who was connected in some way with the Todd lab, and who, discerning me somewhere in the back recesses of the kitchen, recognised me as a familiar face. Somewhat shocked, he asked me what on earth I was doing there. If I wanted a meal job, it should be on campus. It should, moreover, be at the place where Ed himself had a meal job—namely, the Elizabeth Waters Residence Hall, a dormitory for women students. He got me a job immediately, and I continued to be a student employee at 'Liz Waters' for the remaining three years of my tenure as a grad-student at the University of Wisconsin-Madison.

Ed Thorpe's intervention was a gift of high proportion, though I am sure he was unaware of its magnitude; I am equally sure I failed to recognise it or to acknowledge it adequately. For a year or so I scrubbed stoves in the basement kitchen of Liz Waters in return for my dinner, and later loaded dish-washing machines before 'moving up' to the dining-room area. There, as a 'busboy', I was mainly occupied in handling huge oval trays of empty dishes, taking them out to the serving area and sending them on their way downstairs to the basement kitchen. The trays were routinely carried on one shoulder, supported with one hand.

Yes, it had to happen!—though I don't remember it happening to anyone else in my time. One unforgettable evening, the tray slipped. The tray did not suddenly land on the floor. As it tilted, it started to shed its load, and the sound of smashing crockery caught the attention of the young women who were eating their dinners. The big metal tray bounced, clanged and clattered to great effect, making a wonderful din as it hit the hard, ceramic tiles of the floor. I am happy to say that I had the presence of mind to keep walking, without pause and without so much as a backward glance. Once concealed in the serving station, I joined in the merriment and laughter of everyone there. I was not hiding. Lots of people had watched me being overtaken by catastrophe, and I happily (perhaps proudly) joined the throng of colleagues in cleaning up the mess. It was not funny unless you were there of course, and the managers and bookkeepers who were not there could not have been amused when they heard about it. I was not asked to pay reparations, nor did I forfeit any of my meal-job meals. In retrospect, I am impressed by, and very grateful for, the generosity of all concerned.

Eventually I moved right up to the position of waiting on tables. This was, as the saying goes, like dying and going to heaven! Before dinner was served to the residents, all of the male and female student workers would have dinner together, so I spent time every day in the company of young students. Elizabeth Waters Hall had its own dock on the shore of nearby Lake Mendota, and in summer, when our dinner duties were done, we adjourned to the dock for swimming and camaraderie. Sometimes we would organise a picnic or party for the weekend, meeting at some park for beer and hotdogs and that sort of thing. Spending almost all my daytime hours in the laboratory, I welcomed the social fringe-benefits of my evening meal-job. In the end, I think I would have seriously considered working there even if I had to pay the university for the privilege of doing it!

My research studies in Wisconsin were suspended by my return to Ireland in 1954. At some point during that summer, I mentioned to my father that I was cleaning stoves to earn my dinner. I said it with pride. After all, he had made sure that, scholar or not, I had to get up in the morning and shoulder sacks of potatoes and be generally prepared for some honest hands-on labour. My father's reaction to my news was notably cool—no smile of satisfaction, no comment of any kind. I remember being disappointed. I felt 'let down'.

It wasn't until many decades later that I had the thought that perhaps my father, having worked very hard to make sure that his children would not depend on menial labour for their livelihood, got no pleasure from hearing that his grown-up son in a far-away land was scrubbing stoves for his supper. Perhaps it was even something of an embarrassment to him. My disappointment could not, however, even for the moment, make me love my father less. The disappointment had arisen because I loved him so much, and wanted so much to please him. We did not, of course, talk about such matters.

Later, when I was back in Wisconsin, Professor Todd, always looking out for the welfare of his graduate students, handed me an application form for the position of Residence Hall Supervisor. That was a job in which one lived rent-free in a men's dormitory in return for monitoring the behaviour of its undergraduate residents. It was an appealing new idea, so I started filling in the form. Then I got to a question the wording of which was roughly: 'What do you consider your most admirable personal quality?' I stopped right there.

They were, in effect, asking me to say something favourable about myself. They were asking me! I thought of writing in 'modesty' as my answer, but was afraid nobody would see the joke. Stymied, I discarded the form and gave no more thought to the job. The episode was, I suppose, a trivial example of cultural incompatibility between the administrative protocol of a big 'melting-pot' organisation and the sensibility of a student of my reserved background.

On another occasion, Professor Todd came to my rescue with an opportunity for some much-needed cash. On very cold mornings in Madison, my old Dodge car became reluctant to start. I routinely parked it on the street in front of Knapp House where I lived. When the engine became even more recalcitrant, I resorted to disconnecting the battery and carrying it into the house to benefit from indoor warmth overnight. One morning I placed the heavy battery, as usual, on the broad Dodge fender to free my hands for the business of installing and connecting it. Everything was icy, including the fender. The battery smashed on the ground.

A day or so later Professor Todd came into the lab and placed a bare wooden box on the bench in front of me, saying 'Here's your new battery'. He had been to the Sprague-Dawley animal supply company in Madison and had arranged to test a few of their rats for parasites in exchange for a certain amount of cash per rat. The rats were in the wooden box. I examined the rats for parasites, received the money, and treated my old car to a brand-new battery! It's worth repeating: Arlie Todd was ever solicitous for the well-being of his students.

Making friends in Madison

For many of my years doing my PhD in Wisconsin, I lived rent-free in the old Governor's Mansion on the edge of Lake Mendota. I had been awarded a Kemper K. Knapp Fellowship, a grant that enables a group of graduate students from various disciplines to live together in an environment conducive to intellectual 'cross-fertilisation.' It was a rare blessing to get into Knapp House, and it involved being interviewed by a committee. The bonus of getting in was that you became good friends with people in totally different departments—people, for example, from economics, literature and physics. We all lived in one house as people with dissimilar interests but goodwill towards each other. It was a valuable experience, and a major highlight of my University of Wisconsin-Madison years.

I also met new people through my job at the Elizabeth Waters Hall. A great many young university women lived there, and one was likely to bump into 'Liz Waters girls' at any time and any place. I did in fact bump into one in an all-too-literal sense one winter day. Some of my Liz Waters friends had persuaded me to go skiing with them at the Telemark ski area in northern Wisconsin. They gave me a few rudimentary lessons on the art of skiing (or at least the art of climbing up a slope in herring-bone steps) and pointed me downward on the 'beginners slope'. That was a piece of snow-covered land, sloping gently towards the bottom of the mountain and curving leftward to end at a primitive 'rope-tow' where a line of people stood patiently waiting for the opportunity to grab the rope and get pulled to the top of the hill.

Somehow, I managed to stay upright on my skis all the way down to the rope-tow. The people waiting in line gazed at me with mild interest as I coasted very slowly but very constantly toward them. I gazed at them too, but my interest became far from mild when it dawned on me that I had absolutely no idea how to stop. I bumped into a young woman with just enough impact to knock her down in the snow, but not enough to hurt her. She picked herself up with great good humour and a smile of recognition, and introduced herself as one of the girls who lived at Elizabeth Waters Hall. So the episode ended happily; though a romantic sequel might be expected at this point, I must say at once that there was not a sequel of any kind.

It was probably in the same winter that I was prevailed upon to attach my feet to skates. Some of my friends took evident delight in introducing this young foreign student to the full experience of being an American, and a Midwesterner at that. The Liz Waters kitchen crew would sometimes organise a skating outing on a nearby lake. It sounded enticing and I was eager to try everything. I went to a sporting-goods store and gazed at a whole wall of skates—shelf upon shelf in a perplexing profusion of styles and prices. I found a pair that was surprisingly cheap; so I bought them. When I proudly joined my friends on the next skating expedition, they looked puzzled. And then amused. I had bought racing skates. They had very long blades (all the better to speed you along with) and very little, if any, ankle support—if you're such a hot-shot skater, why do you need ankle support? There are many differences between skates and skis. Yet I managed to hit upon one significant similarity. Both of them are hard to bring to a standstill if you don't know how. I didn't knock anyone down on skates, but, for a time, I kept travelling much further in one direction than I wished. I never did buy another pair of skates.

That was not the end of my meal-job fringe-benefits. Still eager to broaden my American experience, I joined my Liz Waters friends in an excursion to the Wisconsin Dells. The Dells are renowned for natural beauty and probably for other things as well, but the one feature that is indelibly marked in my memory is the sandstone massif that fronts a river in a series of cliffs. This time my friends, to give them credit, took the matter of preparation very seriously indeed. One of them, Bill Chipman, had the experience and the wisdom to see that the thing was done properly. They taught me how to install and operate the harness used for rappelling down the face of a cliff.

The harness, as I faintly recall, was linked to a rope that was wound around a tree and held by a member of the group who was delegated to 'belay' the one making the descent. When it was my turn to stand at the edge of the precipice, I turned my back to the void, crouching slightly, and leaned backwards over edge, with just my feet touching the edge and with the rope and harness giving solid support to my body. At once I felt completely confident, assured that all was well. Then the fun part—a series of controlled drops in which you spring away from the cliff face and release the mechanism that allows the harness (and you) to slide down the rope for the short period that you and the rope are away from the cliff. Repeat until you reach the bottom. All you have to do is to remain facing the cliff so that when the rope swings you back to the cliff at the end of each drop, you meet it, not with your back, but with your feet and the cushioning springiness of your legs. It was exhilarating! By some circuitous route, of which I have no recollection, we returned to the top of the cliff and picnicked on a patch of scrubby grass. That night I dreamed about falling, and for the first time (and, I believe, the last time) I was able to connect something weird and scary in a dream to something that had happened during the previous day.

New Jersey
and other parts
of the world

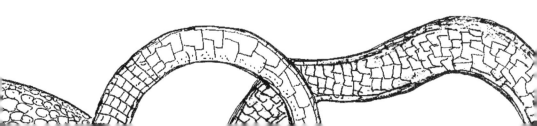

Moving to Merck

It has always been amazing to me how the really big decisions in life are brought about by chance. My going to the United States was entirely because Professor Todd in Wisconsin wrote to Professor Smyth at Trinity. Then at the end of graduate school when I was finishing my PhD, I was applying to colleges assuming I would stay in an academic career. Out of the blue Professor Todd got a letter from Ashton C. Cuckler at Merck & Co. Inc., asking if he had anyone finishing that he would recommend. So Todd, who was unusual in being a very pro-industry professor, suggested me and told me I should go and interview.

I consulted a map and saw that Merck was located in New Jersey amid a big mass of yellow spots—it looked like it was a totally built-up area. This was not appealing to me, and industry certainly was not appealing. But Todd said go and talk to them, convincing me by mentioning that I could visit nearby New York City again while I was there. So I went, and I did go to New York. I went to Broadway and for $8 I saw Charles Lawton starring in George Bernard Shaw's 'Major Barbara'. I sat in an excellent seat just a few rows from the stage. Already the journey had not been wasted.

But then it got even better. I discovered when I actually went to Merck to see Dr Cuckler and his department of parasitology, that it was very, very impressive. My outlook started to change. I went to one of my professors at Wisconsin and asked his advice: if I were to do this industry research for a year would I be so tainted that I could not get back into academia? He said no, no, don't worry about that. So I thought I would give it a try. In March 1957 I started my first job as a professional scientist, employed at the Merck Institute for Therapeutic Research, an institute within Merck. I quickly discovered it was vastly superior to anything I had anticipated. I learned more and I learned faster than I did in graduate school; which is not to put down graduate school. It is, after all, a different environment entirely.

It was so exciting to be in research at Merck where everybody was committed and working towards related goals, and it was a very enjoyable condition in terms of being able to do things that had defined objectives, but also to follow ideas that just occurred to you in research and have the funding available to explore them.

I was extremely lucky too: not all companies are the same, and not every company is the same from one time to another, from one division to another, or from one department head to another. But this company, at this time, with these people suited me perfectly, and I didn't quit after trying it out for a year. Instead I stayed at Merck until I retired, 33 years later!

Announcing new treatments

Experimental chemotherapy, which is mainly about finding new chemicals to treat or prevent disease, is intrinsically exciting, because promising observations are almost sure to be made from time to time. When that happens, the wise experimentalist will be moderate in excitement, because of the plethora of obstacles that face any prospective new drug. When a novel biodynamic substance can be reasonably regarded as a potential new drug, it is customary (and ethically mandatory) to call it to public attention because of its scientific significance—and commercial potential, if any. It is conventional, too, to do that by means of what might be termed 'announcement publications'. Such articles are neither reviews nor abstracts, but first reports of the critical findings in chemistry and biology that constitute discovery of a particular drug. I have had the great good fortune to have shared authorship of six such publications.

Looking back on my experience with drugs that were successfully marketed by Merck, I see a rough sort of pattern. At the beginning of my career there was thiabendazole, a broad-spectrum anti-roundworm agent that set a new standard in the control of livestock parasitism. That was followed by cambendazole, a chemically related compound with enhanced efficacy against tapeworms. In the 'middle' of my career there was the anti-fluke agent rafoxanide (with greater than usual efficacy against young flukes), followed by clorsulon (effective against even younger flukes). Toward the end of my career there was ivermectin (anti-roundworm, anti-arthropod parasites) with numerous applications, including (and of special interest to me) the prevention of canine heartworm disease, and control of river blindness, elephantiasis, and other parasitic infections of humans. Ivermectin, in turn, was followed by the chemically related eprinomectin, developed specifically for use in dairy cattle.

From flatworms to roundworms

Even though the Nobel prize had been awarded largely for science that reduced the burden of river blindness, I never worked directly on that parasitic disease. But that is the beauty of parasitology—by working on the biology of a range of parasites, and with interesting twists and turns along the way, you get insights that can help to tackle a disease caused by a particular parasite.

It will be recalled that when I was at the University of Wisconsin-Madison, I worked on a type of flatworm, a leaf-shaped giant liver fluke that infests sheep, cattle and deer. When I moved to Merck, initially I stayed in flatworm territory. I started carrying out research on schistosomiasis, also known as snail fever, a disease of humans caused by flukes called schistosomes, which live in the bloodstream. These are a big problem in parts of the developing world where the larvae of the worms live in freshwater snails. The snails shed microscopic larvae that swim free in the water and penetrate the skin of humans using the water for fishing or agriculture, or to bathe or to wash clothes.

The resulting disease of schistosomiasis in humans can cause damage to the liver, the gut, the urinary and reproductive tracts, and schistosomiasis is particularly damaging for children, whose growth can be stunted. At Merck I was hired specifically to work on schistosomiasis. My stated objective was to discover new drugs to treat the disease. It was a fabulous research setup, and I was hoping to continue that sort of work for the rest of my life. We had opportunities to bring in experts on schistosomiasis, and to go to meetings in New York, where I became active in the New York Society of Tropical Medicine, eventually becoming its president.

In this period, my colleagues and I discovered an exceptionally potent drug against schistosomiasis. It was really powerful against the immature parasites, and this is important because you want to catch these worms as early as possible in their life cycle. The drug (a phenyl-quinoline) was put through its paces in various animal models, and every time it proved its potency against these little flatworms. But there was a catch: when mice were given the drug the tips of their noses, paws and ears got sunburned! The drug created photosensitivity, meaning the skin would be more susceptible than usual to damage from the sun's rays, and this was obviously not ideal for parts of the world with a lot of sun exposure. So it didn't go through the rounds of clinical trials in humans that would be required to put it on the market. Thanks to the photosensitivity side-effect, our drug never saw the light of day.

I spent seven years at Merck working directly on schistosomiasis, and continued to supervise the project for many subsequent years. I had a totally unblemished record of failure—and I had a ball! It was just wonderful. No one was upset with me, partly because I was publishing and discovering interesting things all the time. I hoped to go on doing it, but one day Dr Cuckler came to see me with a new work proposition that changed my research direction. I was sitting at the microscope, and he put on the bench beside me a damp paper towel and said perhaps I could use this in connection with a new drug that my colleague in the next lab was working on. It turned out that the paper towel had in it the carcass of a mouse with trichinosis (now trichinellosis), a disease caused by parasitic roundworms (not flatworms) called *Trichinella*, and the drug next door was called thiabendazole.

Thiabendazole was to become the first big breakthrough in treating roundworm in sheep and cattle. It was a blockbuster that brought about a whole shift in animal management, partly because, unlike the conventional drugs, it did not cause a setback in the animals' growth after treatment. From then on, I became very interested in working with the trichinosis parasite in the lab and testing drugs against it. And when I tried the drug from the next-door lab, it worked. Thiabendazole killed larval development of the parasite in the muscles. Ultimately it did not find a significant application as a drug for trichinosis in humans, but knowing that it worked was useful nonetheless.

I wrote a whole series of papers on trichinosis, including how the worms find each other to mate in the small intestines of mice, and I eventually edited and co-wrote a text book on Trichinella. That roundworm-infested mouse carcass broke my fixation with flatworm flukes, and, looking back, I realise that biodiversity is a good thing at the lab bench as well as outdoors.

Liver fluke again—at Merck

In my early years at the Merck laboratories, I worked under the leadership of Ashton Cuckler, director of the department of parasitology. He had been trained as a classical parasitologist and had found his perfect niche as an industrial scientist. After I had been in his department for several years, he happily supported my desire to set up a programme for research on the treatment of disease caused by *Fasciola hepatica*, the common liver fluke—which, as previously noted, is a livestock disease of world-wide importance. Having worked with the giant liver fluke in graduate school, I would now have a chance to work on the common liver fluke: a 'classic' parasite of medical and veterinary textbooks. It is the 'flocke' that mediaeval shepherds feared because it caused their lambs to die from 'rotten lyver'. It would be one of the creatures that the Reverend Kirby, in his famous Bridgewater treatise, called 'these unclean and disgusting creatures' that surely could not, in his opinion, have sullied the likes of Adam and Eve. For me it was, in a strange way, an honour to work on the common liver fluke. That would not make it any easier!

For years, I had easily raised the snails that I needed for my work on snail fever (schistosomiasis). They are aquatic and do well in an ordinary 'household' aquarium. The snails that transmit the common liver fluke dwell on wet mud-banks, and I spent quite a lot of time creating indoor 'benchtop' mud-banks. It would not be necessary to reproduce a mud-bank ecosystem in all its complexity of fauna and flora, but it would have to be good enough, and constantly wet enough, to support the propagation of mud-bank snails. Fortunately, word soon began to seep through the scientific community that the flukes would develop quite happily in a certain type of aquatic snail. That made things much easier, though it was still a challenge to maintain the complicated liver fluke life cycle in the lab.

My colleagues and I set up our usual harmonious and symbiotic relationship with our Merck colleagues in organic chemistry, who provided us with materials to test against liver fluke, and developed synthetic protocols in conjunction with our test results. Once the liver-fluke assay procedures were in place, the testing of various chemically synthesised substances for effectiveness against fluke in rats was initiated; that was in May 1965. The efficacy of the compound that would later be named rafoxanide was discovered in September 1966. In October 1967, after demonstration of its safety for use with mammals and exceptional efficacy against immature fluke in sheep, I formally recommended it (jointly with Dale Hoff, the head chemist on the project) for development as a commercial product. Things went well and in 1969 we formally announced the discovery of rafoxanide. After the usual creative period of developmental research, it was launched commercially as Ranide (and other trade names). It was a leader in its field for several years and continued to enjoy a place on the animal-health market for decades. Later, when my responsibilities became broader, Dan Ostlind took over the running of the liver fluke program. The interdepartmental collaborations again succeeded, leading to the announcement of clorsulon in 1977 and its similar success as a veterinary pharmaceutical product (sold commercially as Curatrem, etc.).

In all of our research, emphasis was squarely set on innovation. There is little pride to be had in making 'copycat' discoveries or products. At the same time, science is forever cumulative. Wisps of past discovery permeate the scientific atmosphere. No discovery is entirely lost. The lineage of a discovery is often obscured but is seldom without interest.

Rafoxanide belongs to a broad class of chemicals called salicylanilides (their effect on flukes had first been reported by an Austrian veterinary pharmacologist). Clorsulon belongs to the sulfonamides. It is interesting, I think, to reflect on the fact that the anti-fluke salicylanilides have distant germicidal ancestry, while anti-fluke sulfonamides are relatives of the 'sulfa drugs' once famous in the treatment of pneumonia and other bacterial diseases. That is not to suggest that there is much chemical or pharmacological similarity between the ancestors and the descendants. Within each of those two classes (and between them, as well) there is huge variation in chemical structure and biological properties. As with our own human heritage, there is much to wonder at.

FASCIOLA

Blade of life, leaf aquiver,
Soft and brown, motile sliver,
Blood is pond, bile is river,
Haven safe, deep in liver.

Trespass and forgiveness

Sometimes bad things happen; and sometimes it is somebody else's fault. I am not talking here about truly devastating misfortune. But nor am I talking about trivial things—as for example, when your very young child switches television channels at the very worst moment of live action. No, I am talking about 'in between' things, about 'mildly devastating' situations, and especially about events that bring you a significant hurt under a special circumstance.

In one instance that comes to mind, my actual response surprised me. It relates to my research on the parasitic disease trichinosis. My central interest covered many adventitious sub-topics, including the immune response of animals to the presence of the parasite. One unanswered (and rarely asked) question was: could immunity be evoked by the microscopic life-cycle stage of the parasite known as the 'newborn larva'? In the scientific community at large in the 1960s, lack of interest in the topic had been due primarily to the difficulty in harvesting the larvae in large numbers.

While doing experiments on other aspects of trichinosis, my technicians and I found a way to do that. Here was the chance of a lifetime! We would be the first to introduce newborn larvae into mice in a manner that completely bypassed their normal migratory route within the mammalian body. Would that enable the larvae to elicit an immune response? If so, would the response be the same as, or in addition to, the response elicited by the natural infection?

When I say that we found a way to collect newborn larvae, I do not for a moment mean to imply that we found an easy way. We found a very laborious way—and that is central to this account. Eventually the day came when we had collected enough larvae to do our planned experiment. The delicate creatures, far too small to see with the naked eye, were suspended in saline in a very small beaker; I stood ready, syringe in hand, to inject the designated amount intravenously into our test mice.

It happened in the blink of an eye! One of the technicians brushed a hand against the beaker, knocking it over, spilling the precious liquid onto the bench. There was no way to retrieve our invisible larvae in useable condition. We cleaned things up. No word was spoken. No swearing, no reproach, no apology. We all knew that it was an accident. We knew that we would not do the experiment again. In hindsight, I reproach myself for not scheduling another attempt—but we were busy, and this had been an experiment done 'just for fun' and a digression from things more immediately at hand.

The point, of course, is that the very enormity of the thing was such that I knew instantly and instinctively that anger would be absurd. I did not suppress anger; I claim no credit for restraint; anger simply did not arise. Sometimes, when someone's innocent action causes you great distress, the impulse to anger simply drains away. We can all be glad of that.

Losing father,
meeting Mary and becoming a US citizen

The late 1950s and 1960s marked a period of a profound change in my personal life. My father died, then a few years later I met and married my wife, Mary, and we started our own family.

My father died in 1956. He had been diagnosed with cancer, and he had bouts of treatment. The end came quickly, though, and it was a surprise. I almost didn't find out in time. In the early hours of the morning in Madison, Wisconsin, I received a call from my brother Bert in Donegal, asking why I had not responded to the telegram he had sent. The telegram bore the news that my father was dying and he wanted to see me. But, through human error, that telegram didn't reach me. There was no time to dwell on that, it was imperative that I got home quickly to Ramelton.

With the co-operation of an airline, and with two family friends driving almost the length of Ireland, meeting me at Shannon Airport and rushing back up north through heavy rains, I made it back to the family home. My father managed to speak to me very briefly. He died the next day. He was 74. Just before he passed away, my father's last words were 'I've had a good innings'. It is ironic that the word 'innings' as a singular noun was, as far as we were concerned, a cricket term, and my father was less interested in sports than anyone I have known.

His death, and those of my mother and brothers in later years, naturally created a very deep sense of loss. I go back from time to time, an internal turning back, and realise how much I miss them. That brings a deep sadness, and it will never go away. Soon after my father died, I returned to the USA to continue my scientific work.

A few years later, in 1960, there was a tremendously positive development in family life: I met Mary Mastin. I had had few romances before then, and even back in my college days my social life could be described as subdued. In Trinity College

Dublin, the big social event of the year was the annual Trinity Ball, held at one of the big hotels in downtown Dublin. I remember attending three of them. They were social challenges for me since, unlike Lexie, I never got over the feeling of being behind in the social world of college life.

For the first Trinity Ball, I invited the young woman who sat next to me in my first science classes. She was extremely pretty, and I developed a romance with her that was mostly wishful thinking. She was a Derry girl and she had visited me briefly in Ramelton during summer vacation. I was to re-connect with her late in life, and invited her and her husband to a couple of functions in Dublin—at which her husband was given to teasing his wife by asking her why she had let me get away.

The second Trinity Ball date was a classmate and ex-WAVE (a Royal Navy auxiliary force during World War II), and she was a bit older than I was. We had a friendship, but not a romance. I cannot remember the name of the third, probably because I do not have a photograph taken on that occasion. I sometimes thought enviously of those who experienced a 'grand passion' in their undergraduate years. Finally, in my Wisconsin grad-school days I had a few serious romances, but did not feel ready for marriage.

But when I met Mary I was ready! In Elizabeth, New Jersey, I attended a church that had periodic social 'mixer' events. At one of them, two young women from out of town arrived—and I hit it off with one of them, the lovely Mary Mastin. She had come at the request of a friend, who had an existing interest in a member of the group and wanted Mary to come as her companion. Common at such events were devices to enable, even coerce, young people to share interests and attitudes. Mary and I had some interests that were not those most commonly expressed at church affairs, including drinking and skiing. Perhaps we were being a bit provocative just for fun. The church was liberal in outlook, the people in the group were young, and declarations such as ours were greeted with a laugh, not a frown.

The result was a date at a quiet suburban bar in Ho-Ho-Kus, New Jersey and a decorous sampling of Irish whiskey. We started dating, which meant a lot of driving because we lived about an hour's distance apart—Mary was working as an occupational therapist at a cerebral-palsy center in New Jersey.

After a couple of years of not-always-smooth dating, we were married on 24 February 1962. Two years later, I applied for US citizenship. This was precipitated mostly by the times spent sitting at the lunch table at Merck and getting involved in discussions about civics and politics but feeling uncomfortable because I had no vote, no real say in the game. If I was going to stay in the US, I felt an obligation to become a citizen.

In the early stages of the process I filled out forms in which I declared that, to the best of my knowledge, I was not, and never had been, a member of the Spanish Falangists and that I was not, and never had been, a prostitute. My memories of the process are now faint, but I believe these two declarations are pretty accurate; they were, after all, of a memorable nature. The forms also asked my mother's age, and I thought 'You have some nerve asking that!—and I am not going to ask her'. Fortunately, an answer was not required for that particular question.

In due course, I was interviewed at the courthouse in Elizabeth, New Jersey, by a representative of the Department of Justice of the United States. On his desk, he had a big dossier containing my application and supporting documents. He asked me to confirm that my application was truthful and complete, and I cheerfully assured him that it was. He pointed to the dossier, and with just the tiniest smile of triumph, said that I had been a member of the Dublin University Philosophical Society, but had not recorded that fact in the application. I was floored. It had not occurred to me to mention that bit of trivia. Yes, I had been a member of 'the Phil' at Trinity; it was where I had enjoyed many lively debates and, as mentioned, I had even seen a visiting Éamon de Valera, but how on Earth did the American authorities know that? The examining official was not at all confrontational. I think he just enjoyed the moment. My omission of Trinity Phil membership on the application form was not a problem; at a ceremony on 30 November 1964, I became a US citizen.

By then, we were parents. Mary stopped working during our child-raising years, after which she eased gradually back into the work-force, choosing work opportunities as they accommodated school hours. Among other occupations, she worked as a dental assistant, as an assistant to a ceramics artist, and ended as office manager for a small group of salesmen. Now, after more than a half-century of marriage, we remain very much devoted to each other. We live in what must be our final few years, and the prospect of being without each other's loving support is unthinkable.

Parenthood

In 1963 I crossed the Atlantic Ocean again, this time to England to do some basic parasitological research at Cambridge University. It was exciting enough to be going to Cambridge. It was, after all, a 'gemstone' in the British university system and, moreover, I was going to take up an opportunity to work in the laboratory of E. Lawson Soulsby, later Professor Lord Soulsby, Baron of Swafham Prior.

My work in England would be on the immune response to the *Trichinella* roundworm. In those days, people were greatly surprised by evidence that the immune system could tackle a worm parasite—a pathogen vastly bigger than a bacterium. Lawson Soulsby was a pioneer in the field. We did not work closely together (he was much in demand around the world as a speaker on this 'cutting-edge' immunology) but we became friends. Later, when he was the speaker at a scientific meeting in New Jersey, I had an opportunity to introduce him as 'His Lordship!'

But there was more. I was going with Mary to whom I had been married for only a year—and to cap it all, Mary was pregnant. We would sail to England on the famous liner *Queen Elizabeth*; and Merck would generously pay our fare and continue to pay my salary. How much excitement can one person stand?!

Mary's mother had been taken aback by Mary's announcement that she was off to have her baby on the other side of the ocean. Happily for me, Mary took it all in stride, for she had the spirit of adventure—a spirit that endured as she was to give birth to babies in three different countries.

When the time came for our first baby to be born, Mary was admitted to the Evelyn Nursing Home in Cambridge. This was the place where, we were told, the great physicist Lord Ernest Rutherford had died in 1937. (Rutherford had supervised the research done by my Trinity physics lecturer E.T.S. Walton when he and Cockcroft were doing their Nobel-prize-winning experiments on the disintegration of atoms.) But our interest in the nursing home was in beginnings rather than endings. Jenifer Ann

Campbell was born on the afternoon of 17 September 1963, and I was allowed to see her soon afterward. In what was then an English tradition, we spelled her name with only one 'n' and thereby imposed on her a lifetime of explaining and correcting.

As any parent can attest, there is no way to describe the experience of seeing one's newborn child for the first time. It was awesome—awesome back then, before 'awesome' acquired the casually flippant usage of today. What I remember with particular clarity is dining alone that evening in the crowded restaurant of the Blue Boar Inn in Cambridge. Throughout dinner, I longed to leap up and shout 'I have a daughter! Today, I am a father!' I wanted everyone to know that something very special had happened.

Looking back, more than a half-century later, I wonder what it would have been like had I been among friends that evening. They would have showered me with congratulations and joked and clapped and wished me luck. But they could not have understood the 'awesome' part. The awe is deeply personal—something, I suppose, that the parents alone can share. The news was soon shared with family and friends, with rejoicing all around—and visits from a few graduate students and faculty members from the Soulsby lab. Mary was in the Evelyn Nursing Home for eight days, and benefited from the care and lessons about how to bath a baby, and so on, that were part of the British system.

We wished to have the baby registered as an American citizen, but doing so presented a practical problem—I had not yet become an American citizen so I could not do the registration. There followed a tense episode in which Mary took a train to London, went to the United States consulate, and registered Jenifer's birth. Meanwhile, I sat in our newly acquired Volkswagen Beetle in a train station car-park with Jenifer asleep in her 'carry-cot.' Our baby was breast fed, and I must have felt great anxiety as to whether Mary would get back from London in time for the baby's next meal. Neither of us remembers our making a contingency plan in case things did not work out as scheduled. No such plan was needed, and our memory of the episode has long since been relegated to the 'can't-believe-we-did-that' category.

When Jenifer was 21 days old, she accompanied Mary and me when we flew back to the USA. Fatherhood was on; and it would, I am happy to say, become a lifetime affair.

Becoming a dad also had an unexpected effect: it led me to take up photography. I have often said that I think of my forays into poetry and painting, not as hobbies, but as professional 'extensions', in which I tried to blend my pursuit of the arts and my study of parasites. Photography was different; it was a hobby and it started when I showed a colleague a photograph that I had taken of Jenifer. She was just over one year old and looked (of course) beautiful in her little white dress. But the image was a little blurry. My colleague, himself a keen photographer, asked to see the negative; he pointed out that the image on the drug-store print was not as 'sharp' as in the negative. At his suggestion, I set up a darkroom in our basement and eventually devoted a great many hours to developing and printing black-and-white pictures (occasionally sepia toned) of all kinds of subjects, taken in all kinds of places. They included the picture of Mary in the photo section of this book.

By the mid-1960s, the Lamaze technique was all the rage among those concerned with the end of pregnancy, in what used to be called 'lying-in' or 'confinement', Doctor Lamaze had popularised a method of helping mothers, and fathers too, through that late phase. When we were expecting our second child, Mary and I naturally attended the prescribed series of training sessions. The mother's role, as I vaguely recall it, was largely a matter of deep breathing and blowing. The father's part was ... well, I have no memory at all about that. Looking back to those distant days, my wife suspects that the purpose of the thing was to distract the mother from thinking about the only thing she was thinking about—coping with the throes of labour.

I think the policy at Overlook Hospital in Summit, New Jersey at the time was to allow fathers to attend the birth, where his job was to hold his wife's hand and make what he thought might be encouraging sounds. The truth is that neither Mary nor I have much memory of the labour experience (as seems to be the common experience of our species), but we have instead the unforgettable awareness that on 14 January 1966, our son

Peter DeGray Campbell was born. Again, the birth of a baby was special beyond description, and for a father the birth of a son must touch an emotional chord quite unlike any other.

When Peter was around four years old, he accompanied us to a family gathering in my home town of Ramelton. Once, when he and I were walking hand-in-hand through the town we were greeted with a cheery hello, shouted by someone leaning over a wall on a high terrace across the river. In that very small town the families all knew each other, more or less. I recognised the greeter as member of an auto-repair family, but did not really know this particular man. I shouted back a cheery response and we walked on. Within a step or two, Peter said 'You didn't say "This is my boy Peter".'

I was rocked to my boots by that remark! I realised immediately that as we walked through town I had frequently been stopped by a greeting from people whom I knew only slightly. It was usually a momentary greeting, and I would proudly say 'This is my boy Peter' before moving on. This time I had not done so! I was instantly struck by the thought that Peter was proud to have me introduce him as my son. A cynic will point out that little children always seek attention of any kind, but I will have none of it! I thought then, and I choose to think now, that Peter was proud to have me recognise him as my son. Right or wrong, I walked on with my heart bursting with pride.

In the early 1970s, Mary felt that she would like to experience again the condition of being pregnant, of 'carrying a child' or in biblical words of 'being with child'. She and I agreed that we would very much like to have a third child, but Mary wanted the attendant 'expectancy' as well—and she found it in the Antipodes. We were, at the time, on temporary assignment in New South Wales, Australia. Being pregnant, having two little children to take care of, having a new country (a new continent!) to explore, and being the wife of a busy scientist apt to disappear for weeks to attend meetings on other continents: these are not the makings of a placid unperturbed life, but were fully within Mary's ample supply of courage and enterprising spirit.

As much as possible, we tried to take advantage of opportunities to travel while in Australia. At Jenolan Caves, gatekeepers, quick to spot Mary's expanded girth, would not allow her to descend to the bottom to the deepest cave; nor was she allowed to climb to the top of Ayers Rock (as was generally permissible in those days). But we all got to spend time in many places— including Alice Springs, the Great Barrier Reef, the Blue Mountains, and the marvelous beaches and challenging surf of New South Wales.

In due course, Mary was admitted to the hospital in Liverpool, New South Wales, and on 2 August 1972 Betsy Paterson Campbell was born. No Lamaze program; no eight-day confinement; everything well organised and beautifully executed. Mary, having just turned 40, enjoyed being the subject of interest and surprise to the young mothers around her. The 'awesome' factor was still in force. There is nothing that stirs the heart like the sight of a tiny baby with-tiny-fingernails-and-all, and awareness that there now exists a unique new member of one's own family and of the human family.

Betsy's middle name recalled my mother's maiden name (despite my mis-spelling of it) just as Peter's had been an echo of Mary's mother's maiden name. Being six or more years younger than her siblings, she was welcomed enthusiastically by Jenifer and Peter. Back in New Jersey, Mary's mother was taken aback to receive my telegraphed message that the baby had arrived on a day that had not arrived! It is hard to think of time zones on such occasions. We all returned to the USA in 1973 by way of Perth and the Pacific Ocean. Among our memorabilia is a photograph of our new baby sleeping in an open suitcase on the beach, on the island of Mauritius.

When the children were young, Mary cared for them full time in the home. She was and still is a wonderful mother, and I thoroughly enjoyed playing with the kids. We had endless games on the floor of the living room, hopping around and dancing and rolling marbles and such. It was a lot of fun! Jenifer recalls that I 'used to play silly games with us when we were small, and we loved it. … Dad didn't sing, he never sang. He did love music, though, and he would play Irish music in the house and we would dance around.'

I had only a couple of weeks of vacation each year, and I tried to make as much time as I could to be with my family beyond that. When I became director of parasitology at Merck in 1966, the year that Peter was born, I made an important decision. I decided that from that day on I was not going to take home any work such as writing memos or preparing for meetings. I was influenced by the head of a large financial brokerage firm, I think it was the CEO of Merrill Lynch, who had said that if he had to take work home then either he had too much work to do or he wasn't working hard enough at work. That struck me as sensible and good leadership, so I decided not to take that kind of work home and I stuck to it. If I did writing at home, it would be editing a book or writing a paper that I wanted to publish. I did in the end spend a lot of time doing that, but it was when the kids went to bed. I didn't mind burning the midnight oil for that activity because I like the challenge of writing and it was for my own enjoyment and satisfaction.

Was I different from my own father? In terms of being formal, yes. In retrospect I can see that for me it was a big step to make that transition because I had not inherited a tradition of fathers chatting casually with their children. Fathers were a stern and loving presence; they were willing to play with children on occasion, but never forgot their responsibility for parental guidance. Times had moved on since my own childhood though, and while we were not as overtly demonstrative as perhaps families are today, there was a great deal more friendly interaction and involvement between parents and children than there had been in my own childhood. Today, young families express affection and encourage confidence in children to an even greater extent. So maybe we were part of an ongoing social evolution.

Curiosity froze the worm:
the value of 'tangential' experiments

In 1667 Thomas Sprat of Britain's Royal Society endorsed Francis Bacon's opinion that 'there ought to be experiments of light, as well as of fruit'. Sprat went on to point out that 'in so large and so various an Art as this of Experiments, there are many degrees of usefulness: some may serve for real, and plain benefit, without much delight; some for teaching without apparent profit; some for light now, and for use hereafter; some only for ornament, and curiosity.'

Sometime in the 1950s, I heard a lecture that piqued my interest and that had a lasting impact on my work. The lecture was about attempts to freeze a guinea-pig in liquid nitrogen and bring it back to life. That sort of freezing at very low temperature, known as cryopreservation, had for some time been the subject of dramatic popular demonstrations; it was hailed for its practical utility, such as in the freezing of sperm for artificial insemination in cattle.

It appealed to me as a 'Brave New World' sort of science, and the project described in the lecture was especially visionary. Freezing had been accomplished for cells and a few microscopic single-celled creatures, but the idea of freezing a mammal was considered far beyond the realm of possibility. It wasn't so much a problem of size (although that was problem enough, because of the difficulty of getting protective fluids to all parts of the body simultaneously) but rather a problem of complexity—a mammal's many organs and innumerable tissues would all have to withstand any given freezing process. Just as challenging was the thawing process.

All that made me think about worms. Worms, after all, are bigger than a sperm or an amoeba, but smaller than a mammal. They have a variety of organs and tissues but not nearly so many as a mammal. Wouldn't it be great fun, I thought, to freeze a

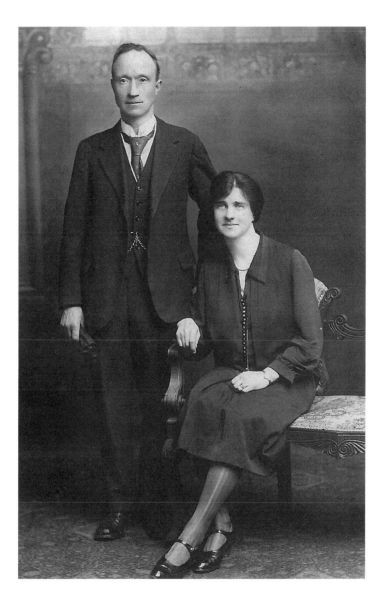

Robert John Campbell and Sarah Jane Patterson Campbell, parents of the author, *c.* 1928.

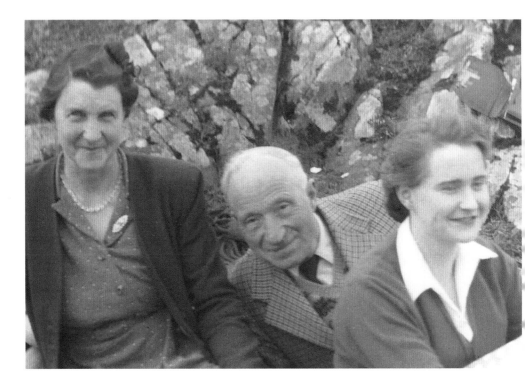

Above: Mother and Father and sister Marion picnicking at Downings, Co. Donegal, August 1954.

Right: Miss Elizabeth L. Martin, tutor to the author and his siblings, *c.* 1940s.

Opposite: Author's Irish passport, 1949, and his Northern Ireland driver's license, 1954.

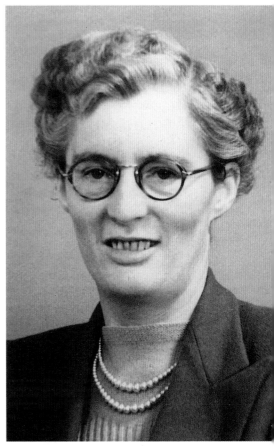

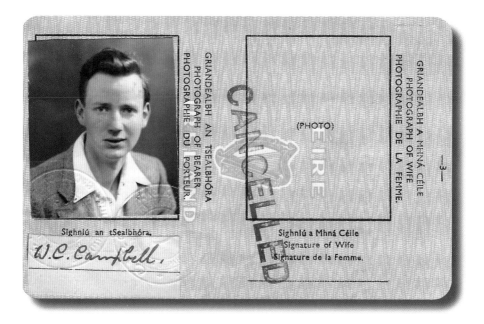

GRIANDEALBH AN tSEALBHÓRA
PHOTOGRAPH OF BEARER
PHOTOGRAPHIE DU PORTEUR.

ÉIRE

(PHOTO)

GRIANDEALBH A MHNÁ CÉILE
PHOTOGRAPH OF WIFE
PHOTOGRAPHIE DE LA FEMME.

—3—

Sighniú an tSealbhóra.

W.C. Campbell.

Sighniú a Mhná Céile
Signature of Wife
Signature de la Femme.

NOT TRANSFERABLE   Licence No. 641934

THE MOTOR VEHICLES

(Traffic and Regulation) Act (Northern Ireland), 1926,
and the Finance (No. 2) Act (Northern Ireland), 1937

**LICENCE to drive a Motor Car of any Class,
including a Motor Cycle**

NOTE—In the case of a Public Service Vehicle a further
licence under Section 12 of the Act of 1926, is necessary

Mr. William C. Campbell

of............Ramelton,

............Co. Donegal.

is hereby licensed to drive a Motor Car for a period of
Twelve Months from the............14th............day of

These pages must not be ren

.............July............19 54 until the............13th
day of............July............19 55 inclusive

RW McIlwaine

Local Taxation Officer

LONDONDERRY

county or County Borough

LONDONDERRY 14 JY 54 LICE

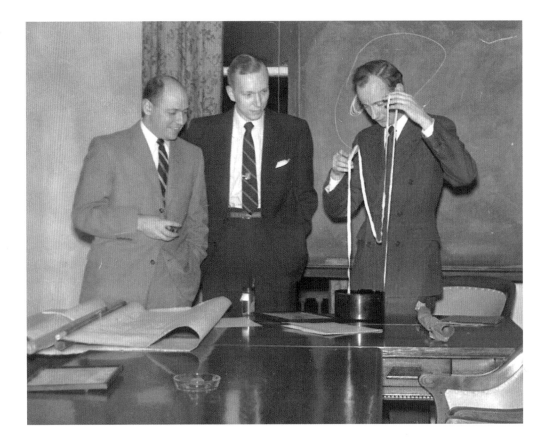

Author demonstrating a tapeworm at Knapp
House, University of Wisconsin-Madison, at the
end of an after-dinner talk, *c.* 1956.

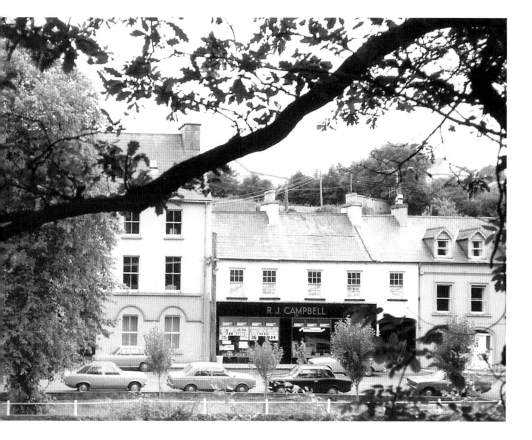

R.J. Campbell's shop on The Mall, Ramelton,
seen from across the Lennon River, probably
1960s. Shop-front modernised from the original.

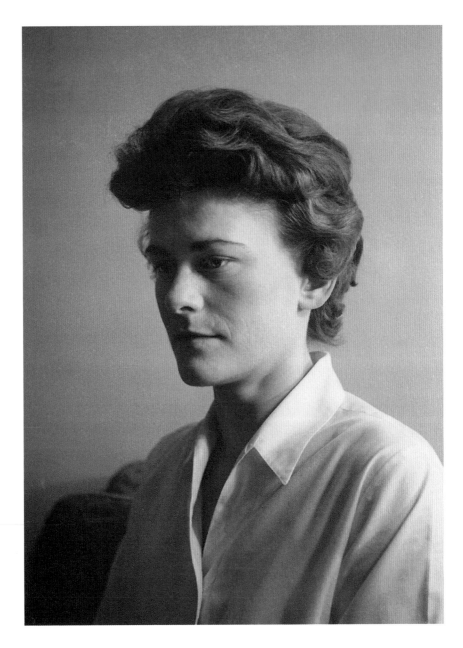

Mary Mastin Campbell *c.* 1961 Photo by the author.

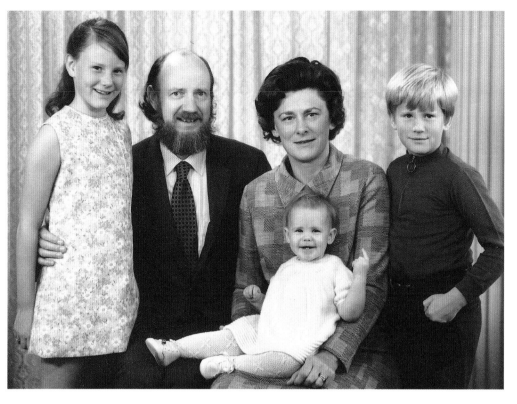

The author and his family in Australia, 1973. Professional photographer not identifiable. Originally published in W.C. Campbell 2016 'Biography', in K. Grandin (ed.), *Nobel Prizes 2015*, 182–95. Nobel Foundation/Watson Publishing International, MA.

Author with his mother and brothers Bert and Lexie in Ramelton, 1960s.

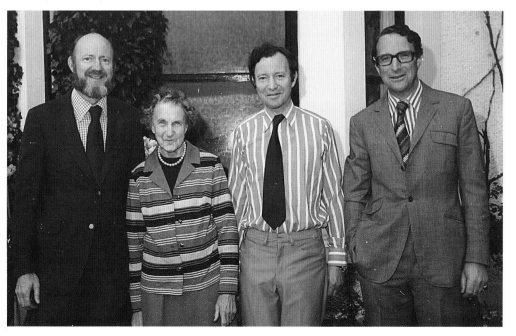

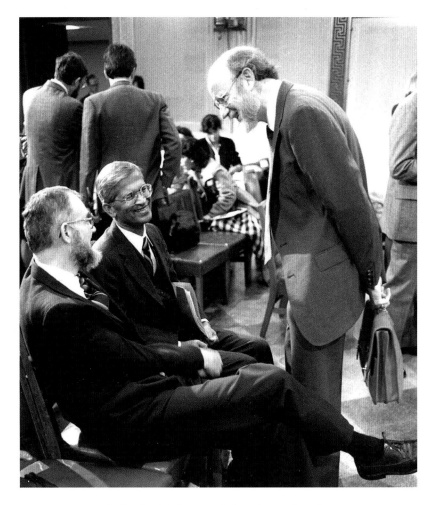

Dr Ken Brown (left), Dr Mohammed Aziz (center) and the author at the meeting at which Merck & Co. Inc. announced its donation of ivermectin for use against river blindness. Washington, D.C., 21 October 1987. © Merck & Co. Inc.; reproduced with permission.

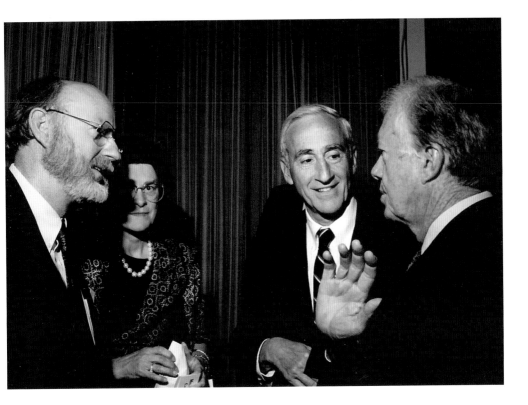

Author and Mary Campbell at the United Nations,
with Roy Vagelos, CEO of Merck & Co. Inc.,
and former US president, Jimmy Carter, 1989.
© Merck & Co. Inc.; reproduced with permission.

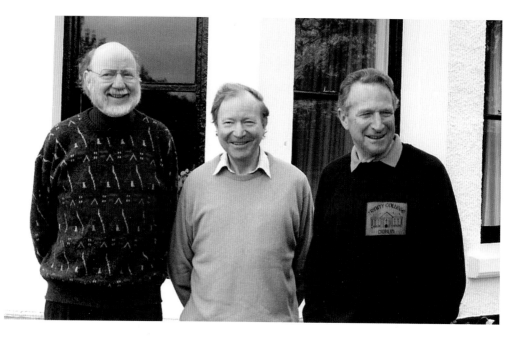

Author with brothers Bert (centre) and Lexie (right), 1980s.

Author with his wife Mary and their three children,
Jenifer (left), Betsy (middle) and Peter (right), 2006.

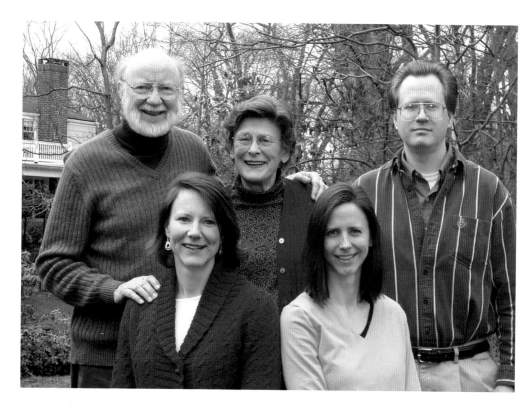

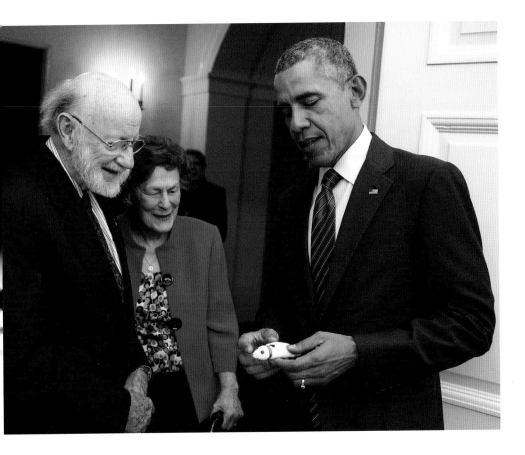

President Barack Obama greets the author and his wife Mary, with gift of toy heartworm. White House, 10 November 2015.

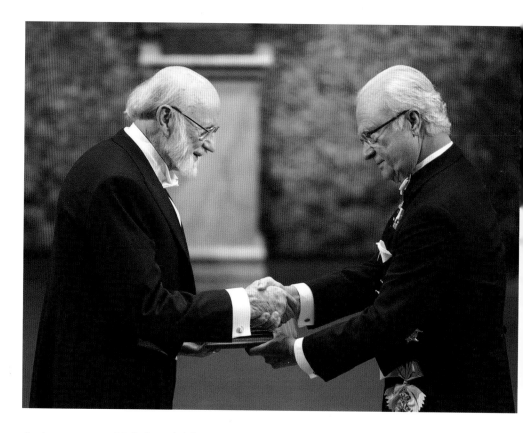

Author receiving Nobel medal from King Carl XVI Gustaf,
Stockholm, 10 December 2015.

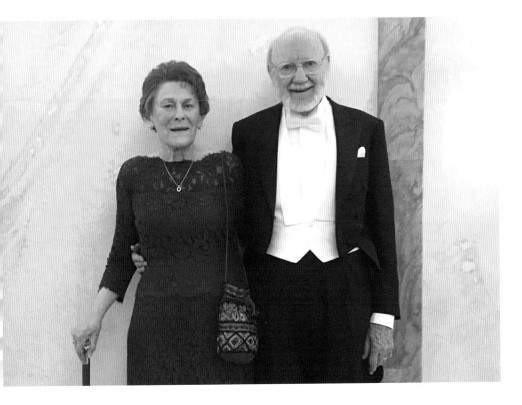

Author and his wife Mary at the Nobel ceremonies, Stockholm, 10 December 2015.

Author and extended family in Stockholm, December 2015. Left to right: Andrew Bluhm, Jenifer Bluhm, Connor Bluhm, Amanda Bluhm, William Campbell, Mary Campbell, Betsy Learner, Adam Learner, Robert Campbell, Anne Campbell.

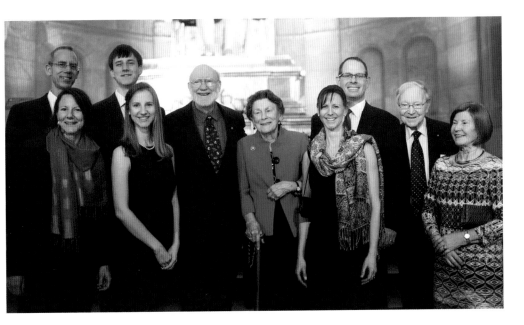

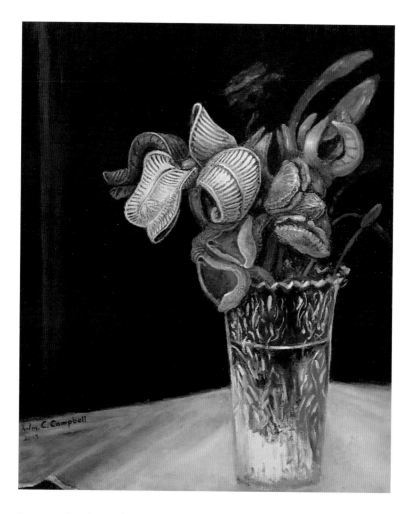

Painting by the author. 'Tapeworms in glass vase';
property of Michael Sukdeo, Rutgers University, New
Brunswick, NJ.

Oil (w.m.) on canvas panel. 2013. *c.* 51 x 41 cm.

Loosely based on: *Rhinebothrium paranaensis,*
Crassuseptum pietrafacei, Paraorygmatobothrium janineae,
Paraorygmatobothrium kirstenae.

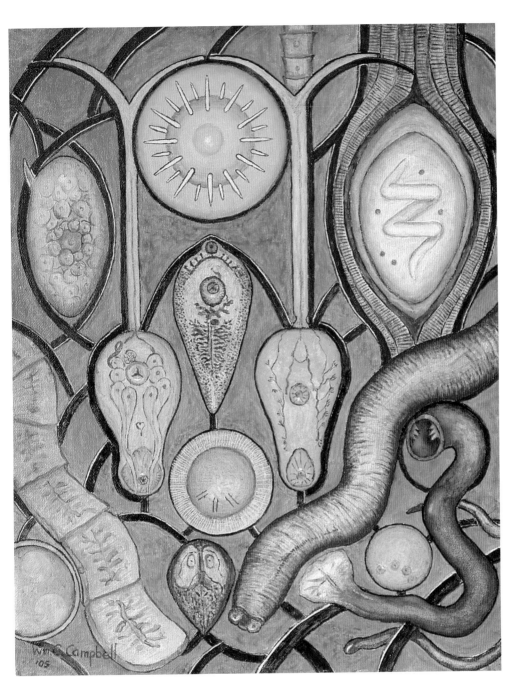

Painting by the author. 'Parasite Window 2'; property
of Stephen G. Kayes, University of South Alabama
College of Medicine, Mobile, AL.

Oil on canvas panel. 2005. *c.* 45 x 28 cm

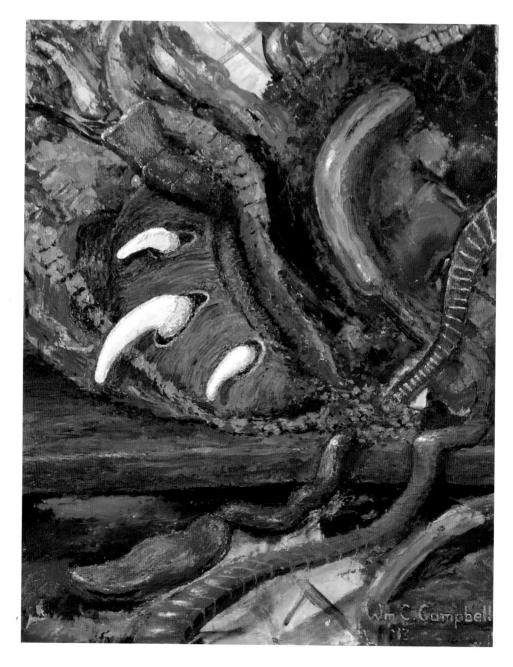

Painting by the author. 'Tapeworms on a shelf';
property of Kelli Sapp, Highpoint University,
High Point NC.

Oil, knife on canvas panel. 2013. *c.* 51 x 41 cm.

worm and, against all odds, have it survive both the freezing and the thawing? So I set about doing it.

The worms selected for my experiments were small. Even within the category of small parasitic worms there are many different kinds—many species of roundworms, flukes and tapeworms. But there was only a handful that I could readily get my hands on. I tried to freeze the species I had in my lab or that were otherwise easily obtainable. The more I tried, the more I failed—and the more I failed, the more I wanted to succeed.

It became a passion. It was not an obsession, because I naturally gave priority to my regular work. I did not think about the possible utility of freezing worms. I thought about becoming the first person to deep-freeze a worm without harming it. My small worms were visible to the naked eye but more effectively examined under a low-power ('dissecting') microscope. I would take worms of a particular kind and freeze batches of them under different conditions. For the most part, this meant immersing them in various protective fluids (cryoprotectants) such as glycerol, and placing the container of worms in a liquid-nitrogen freezer. Later, when I looked at the worms under the microscope I would see a sea of dead worms. No need to count them. They were uniformly and conspicuously defunct.

On one occasion, my assistant, Lyndia Slayton Blair, came back from a coffee-break at Dr Egerton's lab and brought with her a present—a kind of worm known as a trichostrongyle. I put a batch of them through my freezing procedure, and when I looked into the microscope I saw what I expected to see—an expanse of dead worms. But before I raised my head from the microscope, I saw something very unusual. In the midst of that carpet of corpses a few worms twitched! Again, there was no need to count. Whatever the actual account might be, clearly 99.9 percent of the worms were dead. The point, though—the incredibly exciting point—was that the mortality rate was not quite 100 percent!

The worms in this case were larvae of the trichostrongyle roundworm *Haemonchus contortus*. The larvae were at a stage of development in which they are covered with a delicate outer membrane, or 'sheath' that is easily shed under certain conditions. I suspected that the freezing procedure had caused most of the larvae to lose these 'coats,' and that the few survivors had been protected from the cold by keeping their coats on.

Before considering whether it might be possible to freeze larvae by coating them with some sort of artificial outer membrane, there was something else to be done. I took another batch of *H. contortus* larvae and subjected them to a bath in very mild bleach—a procedure known to cause all such larvae to lose their outer coat. My expectation was that this time the picture would be very different—the larvae would all be vulnerable, and I would see, not 99.9 percent dead, but 100 percent dead. Imagine my surprise when I saw that almost all the larvae were alive! My surmise had been completely backwards.

After that it was straightforward. No cryoprotectant was needed! Lyndia Blair followed up with experiments using various rates of freezing and thawing. Remarkably, successful cryopreservation did not require any specialised rate. All one had to do was to place an aqueous suspension of exsheathed larvae in a small screw-cap vial and suspend the vial in the vapour phase of a conventional liquid-nitrogen tank. To thaw the worms, one had only to drop the vial into warm water. (Standing back, in case warm water had seeped under the cap, causing an explosive rate of thawing.) The new freezing protocol worked well for several species of trichostrongyle roundworm. Working with colleagues in Australia and the US, we found that the larvae would survive, and remain infective to other animals, even after cryopreservation for 44 weeks. Eventually Robert Rew and I showed that they were 'as good as new' after 10 years in a liquid-nitrogen freezer. That, I believe, was the longest experiment of my career.

I reported this in 1972, and it has since been adopted as a standard technique. It was gratifying to find that the exsheathment method of deep-freezing worms was of great value to scientists conducting research on trichostrongyle roundworms—though not other types of roundworm. Without cryopreservation, it was necessary to maintain various species and strains of trichostrongyle worms by repeatedly infecting animals—usually sheep or cattle rather than lab-animals. This new method avoided the huge financial costs for large-animal facilities and technical and nontechnical staff. Now, thanks to the success of the method, researchers could establish a 'worm bank' to suit their requirements.

Some years later, in 1978, my colleagues and I overcame a major obstacle to doing research on 'filarial' worms. These make up a large group of parasites, some of which cause diseases in humans, livestock and other animals. We found that such worms grew happily in ferrets, which are relatively easy to work with in the lab environment. The use of ferrets went on to play an important role in the development of ivermectin (in the commercial form HeartgardR) as the first once-a-month medication for the prevention of heartworm disease in dogs. Other lab animals are now used in research on filarial worms.

This kind of 'tangential' experiment on techniques and methods might not be glamorous or catch the headlines in the way that drug discovery or clinical trials can do. But sometimes focussing on the process leads to more outwardly obvious advances.

Getting under the skin of exotic diseases

Parasitic diseases are very satisfying—not to have, of course, but to study in the lab. I have been fortunate also in being able to study diseases of people and domestic animals without the distress of sharing or confronting the pain of the patient. Even better, though hard to bring about, is to experience an occasional 'reality check' in which to observe actual human patients, and to do so, not as the responsible medical clinician, but as an on-site observer.

That is what the Inter-American Fellowship in Tropical Medicine was all about. Run by the Louisiana State University, it was initially restricted to physician participants. Eventually it was opened up to non-physicians and (later still) to industrial scientists like me. As a result, in 1966 I had the benefit of visiting many hospitals and clinics in Central and South America.

Of special note was a visit to the dermatology clinic of Dr Francisco Battistini, in a small village on the banks of the Orinoco River in Venezuela. On the morning when I (and four companion Fellows) visited Dr Battistini, he was treating a boy of about ten who was suffering from Cutaneous Larva Migrans (CLM), more commonly, and meaningfully, known as Creeping Eruption. It is caused by immature dog hookworms that invade the skin of humans. Because people are 'unnatural' hosts for the species of hookworm that occurs in dogs, development into adult worms does not occur. The immature (larval) stage, however, provokes a painful rash and itch.

It happened that we had developed thiabendazole in our laboratories at Merck, and it was being widely used in veterinary medicine for the control of nematode worms. Fortunately, it had recently been introduced into human medicine. One of its special veterinary advantages was its efficacy against larval stages of nematode worms dwelling in tissues outside the intestinal tract. Orville Stone in Texas had reported some preliminary data indicating that this would apply also to human medicine—thiabendazole was effective in CLM!

I mentioned this to Dr Battistini, but he did not seem interested. That afternoon, he took us fishing in a small motor-boat on the Orinoco River. It was hinted that we were fishing for piraña. Whatever sort of fish we were after, we did not catch any; perhaps that was just as well. The boat was idling on the river in bright sunshine, and in that relaxed atmosphere I again brought up the subject of thiabendazole, as tactfully as I could—keeping in mind that I was there to learn not to teach. Again, no response.

Months later, it turned out that Dr Battistini, astute physician that he was, had been listening quietly and stowing away information that might prove useful. He wrote to tell me that his region was getting a lot of rain, resulting, in turn, in a lot of damp, sandy soil in which hookworm larvae thrive, resulting in a lot of Creeping Eruption. He inquired about the name of the medication I had mentioned during my visit, and requested a sample. I was happy to comply; Dr Battistini subsequently published one of the first papers on the efficacy of thiabendazole in Creeping Eruption.

It was an instructive case, in that the Creeping Eruption was on the cheek of a baby, and the case had been complicated (as is common) by secondary bacterial infection. For years thereafter, when lecturing to students I used to show Dr Battistini's photographs of the baby (before and after treatment) to remind them that the value of effective drug treatment can be appreciated only by taking into consideration the distress caused by the intense skin-itch not only to the baby but to its family. Furthermore, apart from the disappearance of the roundworm and bacterial infections, the healing of the damaged skin was impressively fast.

This was one of several observations made by clinicians suggesting that something more than anti-worm efficacy might be going on. I consulted with Merck pharmacologist C.G. Van Arman on this point, and he explored some possibilities experimentally. Together we reported (and got a patent for) the anti-inflammatory property of thiabendazole. That was not the only skin disease to be transformed by modern antiparasitic medication. Ivermectin, much later, proved to be highly effective in the treatment of scabies, especially the previously intractable form known as Norwegian Scabies.

A career setback, Meryl Streep's Dad and a move to heartworm

In January 1972 I took up an appointment as director of the Merck Sharp & Dohme Veterinary Research and Development Laboratory (VRDL) in Campbelltown in New South Wales, Australia. It was a short-term appointment, an exchange between the sitting VRDL director and me, and thus entailed the simultaneous appointment of the VRDL director to my position as director of basic parasitology in the Merck laboratories in Rahway, New Jersey. The arrangement remained in force until Spring 1973, at which time arrangements were being made for the two of us to return to our previous places and roles.

Trouble began when conflict arose between the director who had moved from Australia to New Jersey and the Merck Sharp & Dohme senior management in Australia. In the face of irreconcilable difference, the Australian's return transfer to his Australia post was blocked, so he would stay in New Jersey. I was informed that, on my return to Rahway, I would report to him. He would continue to occupy 'my' office, with the support of 'my' departmental secretary. He would have my old job, while I would be switched, at least figuratively, from the 'executive ladder' at Merck to the 'scientific ladder.'

The 'scientific ladder' is a nebulous concept; it carries little responsibility, respect or security. I protested the proposed plan. While still at Campbelltown, I argued my case in an hour-long phone conversation with the relevant vice president in the Rahway laboratories. In those days, an international phone call of that length was, in itself, highly unusual—as, indeed, was an hour-long argument with a vice president!

On my return to New Jersey, I renewed my protest. The important point was not the indignity of the situation—I doubt if that was ever mentioned—but rather my conviction that, given the personalities of the individual departmental members and leaders, and the complexities of the scientific program, the new arrangement simply would not work in practice. I was told that the rules did not permit a re-structuring of reporting relationships in a way that would accommodate my request to avoid reporting to the person who was sitting in 'my job'. I was told to go and see the head of Human Resources, Harry Streep, and get confirmation of the rule. So, I went and talked to Meryl's Dad. He assured me that the rules imposed no such restriction. It made no difference.

I could have spent more energy trying to resolve this situation, but instead I guess I figured things wouldn't change in the short term, and I found consolation in the fact that I now had the opportunity, with my assistant Lyndia Blair, to focus on basic research in parasitology. This career 'setback' gave me the opportunity to inaugurate a programme on canine heartworm disease, which subsequently gave me the further opportunity to investigate ivermectin as a treatment to prevent the disease in dogs. The dog heartworm is a 'filarial' species of roundworm, as also is the river blindness parasite—so this research foreshadowed the work that would soon be done on the prevention of that disease in humans (and would ultimately be recognised in the awarding of a Nobel prize.) While I could not have known it at the time, perhaps this interlude was less of a career crash and more of an important period of regrouping and getting back to the laboratory bench.

The 'setback' ended when I received a phone call at home one weekend at the end of 1976. It was my boss, Dr Birnbaum, asking if I would be willing to re-assume administrative responsibility for one of the PhD scientists in the parasitology department, owing to what I will politely refer to as an incompatibility between himself and the new director. Eventually, I was asked to assume administrative responsibility for the whole department and to re-assume my position as 'Director of Basic Parasitology'. My office and my secretary were restored to me.

My advice now to anyone who feels they have been thwarted or derailed, is to get back to what interests them in whatever capacity they can, because then at least there will be a source of satisfaction rather than frustration, and who knows what might arise from it.

The smoking memo

In 1968 I wrote a protest memo. Considering my diffidence toward senior Merck personnel, this was not typical behavior on my part—but I did not hesitate to speak out when I thought it important to do so. It this case, the trigger was spending a day at a high-level meeting at our Branchburg Farm conference locale during which the smoking of cigarettes and cigars was more or less constant.

My memo began with the assertion that, for a group of people whose day-to-day activities were directly or indirectly related to matters of health, conditions in the conference room seemed difficult to defend. I went on to propose the prohibition of smoking during conferences (except for routine coffee/tea breaks). I pointed out that experience in factories, churches, theatres, etc., had shown that people are willing to forgo smoking for periods of 1 to 2 hours, and that those whose need to smoke became great in the course of a conference could easily excuse themselves from the room—just as they already excused themselves to answer other irresistible needs.

I foresaw no objections to my proposal in terms of the curtailment of human rights or civil liberties, especially in view of the discomfort endured by the non-smoker under existing conditions, and also because my proposal would not apply to conferences held in individual offices. The health aspect of the proposal would, I argued, present a timely opportunity for the company to make a decree for the benefit of smokers and non-smokers alike. At a time when drastic measures were being proposed elsewhere for the reduction of smoking, I believed it would be entirely appropriate for a health-oriented company like Merck to take a relatively modest but highly symbolic step in that direction. Such a move, I suggested, should not be made quietly or shyly—it should be loudly proclaimed as further evidence that the company was a leader in the promotion of health.

To make sure that my memo would not be written in anger and would not seem to be a 'crank' complaint, I waited for two months after the conference before drafting it. For the same reason I wrote it in a light-hearted, but perhaps too flippant, tone. I am not sure whether it was the tone or the content that caused the head of Merck research, Max Tishler, to suggest to my boss Dr Cuckler that he invite me to withdraw my memo on the ground that it was 'not the kind of document that would sit well in the archives'. Tischler's judgment about that may have been perfectly sound, as it was about practically everything else. Seen in retrospect, however, my proposal did not go nearly far enough. It now appears to have been ahead of its time; 1968, however, was not its time.

In any case, I am glad that I declined to withdraw my memo. Its tone may indeed have been inappropriate in a business setting, but it was prescient! Interestingly, in 2004 my native Ireland became the first country to ban smoking in the workplace, a move that, in Ireland alone, has spared thousands from an early death from respiratory and cardiovascular illness. Today, smoking bans in workplaces are not especially remarkable.

Attitudes and changes

Looking back, I see that my life has had moments of big change. Going to boarding school and going to college were big adventures, but belonged to a more-or-less set pattern. Recreational travel in youth, and subsequent recreational and work-related travel around the world were adventures and decisions of my own making (even those that had been prompted by others). They were new things to do, and as I got older, I saw them as things I knew I could look back on and tell people about. Certainly the biggest, and most fateful, move was my going to America in 1953. Prompted by a professor and intended to last for one year, it was a change that turned into an adventure far beyond anything I envisioned when I crossed the Atlantic Ocean, relatively fresh out of Trinity College Dublin.

In that move, something changed. As I made my life in America, my diffidence dimmed. I was the boy from Donegal, but I was a little wiser now about other parts of the world too, and my confidence grew. My studies, work and social life were positive, enriching experiences and I had a lot of fun with people in this new and different world.

Some aspects of life, however, remained as bedrock, or perhaps as friendly ghosts from my upbringing, and I am glad they hung around. When we were growing up in Ramelton, we were taught that grown-ups were to be respected, and their authority was not to be questioned. We children were also exceedingly polite, and if asked how we were we would reply 'very well thank you'. Even when I was half dead with pneumonia as a child, when asked by my parents or medical carers how I felt, I would reflexively reply 'very well thank you'!

But back to adulthood, I think my admiration for my academic superiors and my managers at Merck drew from that childhood rule about respecting and being polite to those in charge. Some of my colleagues would habitually bemoan 'management' at all levels (and the government). They were 'agin' every sort of authority. I just couldn't see it that way. I thought, and still do think, that the people I worked for were brilliant.

I was often critical of individuals and their actions, of course, and I spoke up for myself when needed. On the other hand, I never felt that I was in constant opposition to some controlling authority. The enduring attitude of respect that was so ingrained in me from childhood probably made it easier for me to work with management rather than 'agin' them.

Science and the arts

While I was working at Merck, I developed an interest in painting as recreation, and ultimately as an expression of my scientific interest in parasites. This didn't come out of the blue. As a student of zoology in Trinity, I would draw complex diagrams of skeletal and anatomical structures—it was certainly how I committed to memory the bones of the gannet and the skull of the Tasmanian devil. I even drew little cartoons with jokes about evolution, ones that played on words; perhaps this was an indication that I was developing some skill in the area, and it was just fun. I am amazed that I used to spend time doing all that drawing just for my own purpose, not to turn it into anything in particular, but to help me build a more complete mental picture of the systems and topics I was learning.

I also drew cartoons and sketches to advertise upcoming events. I did posters for the Dixon Hop, which was a popular dance held in Dixon Hall at Trinity. For one, I copied a Walt Disney illustration of Peg-Leg Pete the Pirate. I drew these posters by hand, painted them with poster paint, and would then add them to the display area by the front gate where students would see them as they entered into Front Square. I was quite pleased when 'my' posters were stolen quickly; it was a mark of their wide appeal!

Now, living in New Jersey, I rediscovered the fun of painting. I had started dating Mary by then, it was around 1960. She was then, and still is, a talented artist. I was living in an apartment with two engineers for Exxon (or Esso as it was at the time), and one of them developed an interest in learning to paint. He suggested that we go to a particular shop in Elizabeth, New Jersey and buy some paints. That appealed to me right away, so we went and got a set of paints from the store and came back to the apartment and started painting. My early paintings had no particular theme; I just started painting copies of other works and pictures by artists such as Van Gogh and Picasso, and they got more and more ambitious over time. Eventually my flatmate and I decided we could exhibit our works at a Greenwich Village Art show in New York City. Some weeks before the show opened, we went to New York to get approval to participate. We had to go in front of the official in charge of the show, who took a quick look at our paintings, checked us off in a book, and allotted us a piece of New York pavement. On show weekends we would bring folding chairs to our spot and display our paintings. We didn't sell anything but one person took an interest in one of my paintings. It was one that I was planning to give to Mary, so I said it wasn't for sale. We still have that painting.

Though I was experimenting with different techniques, my painting continued for a while to lack a theme, and thus to lack passion or purpose. That all changed in 2002, when the American Society of Parasitologists started to have auctions at their annual meetings, to raise funds to support the work of the society. I decided I would do a painting of parasites to help the cause. It was a weird conception of a 'worm monster' featuring schistosome eggs and liver flukes and tapeworms. I had grave misgivings about putting the painting up for auction, because I thought perhaps nobody would bid on it. Though I was apprehensive about that, I went to the auction anyway. Fortunately, a Korean scientist bought my painting, and that really gave me an impetus to paint more parasites as a way to raise further funds for the society. Years later, at another parasitology meeting, I was sitting beside another Korean scientist and we got chatting. Before long we figured out that it was his brother who had bought my painting back in 2002, and he told me the painting was now hanging over the entrance to the owner's clinic in Seoul. That was gratifying to hear.

Since then, I have painted many interpretations of parasites, incorporating their shapes and stages into the works, and sometimes representing them as objects such as flowers or stained-glass windows or Celtic motifs. I use imagination with the colours, because in nature the parasites tend not to be colourful. But they inspire me with their shapes, and with features such as fearsome hooked teeth, visible only by microscope. I paint for fun, and enjoy being able to meld my scientific knowledge and observation with the unconstrained imagination and expression of art. Many of my paintings have raised funds for charities. I jokingly say that my paintings hang in the Natural History Museums of New York and London. I immediately qualify this by pointing out that they hang in the offices of people who work there.

For a while, acting also played a role in my life outside work. I don't know where it came from. As a child, I would play-act with my boyhood friends as so many children do, and at school in Campbell College I had a small part in a production of Macbeth. Yet I had no wish to actually go on stage.

I had not been drawn to acting as a university student, but the church that Mary and I now attended had a programme called The Illuminators, in which little theatrical pieces would be performed, and I took part in many of them. I got the acting bug more seriously when, for some reason, I knocked on the door of a community playhouse in Summit, New Jersey. It was a serious playhouse, one of the longest-running in the Eastern US, having been started in 1918. The woman who answered my knock and welcomed me inside was Betty Kauss, and I saw they were rehearsing for a play. She invited me to come back for try-outs for another play, and I thought what the heck. I tried out for 'The deadly game'. It was a relatively easy role: I played the part of the hangman, which required a lot of sitting on a chair pretending to be asleep. That started me off, and I kept going back and getting bigger and bigger roles, and getting called in to a couple of other playhouses.

Some roles were unexpected too. The Foothills Playhouse, a serious playhouse with occasional semi-professional actors, was staging 'The waltz of the toreadors' by the playwright Jean Anouilh. It was a very successful play in its day. The lead character is a retired French general. The man who was preparing to play that role had a heart attack, and the playhouse called me ten days before the dress rehearsal, about eleven to thirteen days before opening night, and asked me to step in. So I did. I think I was a little hysterical about it. I had to juggle it with my job—I was heading up the biggest department in the Merck Institute at that time—and obviously rehearsals needed to fit in with family life.

There was a huge sense of tenseness and pressure. The last time I could remember being like that was the night before my final exams in Trinity when I went to the movies two times in one day and my roommates told me my language was something else entirely. But, as with my final exams, my dread turned out to have been excessive. Why did I put so much time and effort into acting? I think it was the fun of venturing into an entirely new social milieu. Perhaps it was an ego trip in 'foreign territory'—or maybe it was just an outlet for energy.

In later years, when I lectured to students, I said that science and art are profoundly different, but that what they have in common is creativity. The word 'creativity' is often made to sound rather grand and special. But it is something we all had when we were little kids. The trick is to hang onto it. I encouraged the students to cling to whatever interests they may have in the arts. In my own case, dabbling now and then in poetry and painting may have led naturally to keeping those interests alive.

I would remind the students that many people have worked at jobs of different type. Writers and actors have famously held mundane day-jobs to earn a living. I have (alas!) only a limited and much-neglected affinity with the world of music. Still, I am delighted to know that composer Phillip Glass is an accomplished plumber. Many scientists and other technical people engage in the arts a hobby—as a way of taking a break, as an escape from the heavy demands of their main work. Others develop a more-or-less equally serious interest in both and participate actively in the arts. A Russian chemistry professor was passionate about composing music; now we remember Alexander Borodin, not for his chemistry (or his advocacy of medical education for women), but for his music. In all these cases, science and art are kept separate. This is wonderfully exemplified in the case of Anton Chekov. He considered that working as a family doctor was akin to having a lawful wedded wife; whereas writing plays and humorous sketches was more like having a mistress. So, he said, he tried to keep them as far apart as possible.

I didn't, and still don't, want to keep my science apart from my art. I am under no illusion as to the fact that my involvement is professional in one sphere and strictly amateur in the other. But I don't want to escape from my parasites. I want to bring them with me—into the pictures I paint, into the poems I write. My interest is in combining, or at least blending, science and art. It is an outlook that I recommend.

Keep notes!

Young scientists are told to keep a notebook in which they will record their trials and errors in the laboratory. It should be kept faithfully, recording activities great and small, even calculations that might later be found to have been mistaken. This is sound advice, but I did not always follow it. Throughout my career, I was much given to playing about with things in the lab. Much of what I did would hardly merit the label 'experiment.' Besides, memory is of little concern to the young. Those are my excuses; I was reminded of them (and how hollow they are) late in life— when I realised that I was in possession of a biological image that appeared to be unique. Indeed, when I sent the image to the senior editor of a major parasitology textbook, he inserted it in the next edition as the frontispiece!

What it amounted to was a photograph of the branched intestine of a parasitic worm. In this worm, our old friend the giant liver fluke of deer (*Fascioloides magna*), the extensive intricate branching of the intestine is not fully visible with standard microscopic techniques. Each tiny branch is packed with hematin—an opaque black breakdown product of haemoglobin (presumably acquired from the blood of a host deer or other mammal in which the parasite lives). My surprising new image arose from my attempts to use standard 'clearing agents' to make the tissues of the fluke body transparent and therefore more amenable to microscopical examination. What I found was a way to clear everything in the fluke body except the hematin pigment. I then used a photographic enlarger (without camera or film) to make an image of the entire fluke body in which essentially nothing could be seen except the black hematin, which in turn revealed the distribution of the intestinal branches.

There was a problem! It became apparent only late in life. I discovered that I had no recollection of the methodological trick that had enabled me to make that image. I have been hoping now for a good many years that I would remember how I 'cleared' specimens of that fluke species. The bad news arising from this episode is that, unless that memory returns (and returns soon!) the clearing technique will be lost to science. The good news, as I think about it more than half a century later, is that (as far as I know) the technique is of no earthly use to anyone.

But the unfollowed advice remains solid: keep notes—you never know when you might need to go back to them.

Lessons from the discovery of ivermectin

One of the most important things to note about the success of ivermectin, a primary factor in the awarding of the 2015 Nobel prize in Physiology or Medicine, is that it involved hundreds of people: microbiologists, parasitologists, veterinarians, chemists, lab technicians, experts in clinical trials, people who understood drug distribution in resource-poor settings and of course the executives at Merck who decided to make the medicine available for free to those who could benefit from its impact on river blindness. I was but one of those people involved in ivermectin's success.

Its saga as a therapeutic agent started with a microbe and a mouse. The microbe was from a soil sample that had been collected and examined at the Kitasato Institute in Japan. Soil teems with microbes, tiny bacteria, fungi and other organisms that are invisible to the naked eye. Many of these microbes produce substances that can be useful in some way for humans, such as killing agents that cause disease.

At the Kitasato Institute lab in Tokyo, biochemist Satoshi Ōmura, who shared the 2015 Nobel prize, collected samples of soil from various locations. He and his colleagues then isolated microbes from the samples and looked to see if the microbes had any interesting anti-bacterial activity under 'test-tube' conditions in the laboratory. They also had an arrangement that if microbes were isolated that looked different or had unusual characteristics but were not of direct interest to them, they would send these microbes to Merck Research. Professor Ōmura, who kept a plastic bag with him in case he spotted interesting places to collect soil, had scooped this particular soil sample from close to a golf course near the institute where he worked. That is how a particular kind of microbe, one of many, came from Professor Ōmura's lab to the Merck Research labs in New Jersey, where I worked.

The microbe was then studied by Merck bacteriologists and parasitologists. It was cultivated in laboratory broth, and the broth, after freeze-drying, was added to the food given to a

110

mouse in our laboratories. This was part of a Merck experimental protocol, in which a mouse would be infected with a parasite and then a dried microbial broth would be given to it as part of its regular chow. The mouse would then be examined to see if there was any effect on its parasites. In this case, the parasite that had been used to infect the mouse was a species of roundworm; and when the microbial broth had been added to its food, the roundworms could no longer be found.

This was interesting, of course, but it was not a eureka moment. We had learned not to get too excited by an early result like this, because there are a lot of hurdles that a potential drug needs to overcome before it becomes useful in treating disease in the clinic. This sort of initial sign of interest is near the beginning of that process. In this case, the mouse had almost died before the parasites in it had been killed, and that tempered our enthusiasm at the time too. We later found out that the broth contained a separate substance that was toxic to the mouse, and once this substance was eliminated, the refined broth was safer.

So overall there was subdued enthusiasm at the start, but as the exploration of this microbial broth went on, it kept overcoming the hurdles and my enthusiasm became more overt. It was still guarded though, because even if something makes it through much of the way, it could fall short of being useful as a drug. Even if it is effective for the desired target, there are plenty of potential adverse features, such as being linked to birth defects or other adverse side effects, smelling really bad, or not being chemically stable, and so not suitable for the clinic.

In the case of this particular broth, the extraordinary potency against parasitic worms was what aroused the initial interest. What could be behind it? The microbiologists at Merck very cleverly used a technique to separate out the components of the fermented broth that showed activity against the worm in the mouse. They found that the microbe in the broth was a previously unknown type of *Streptomyces* bacterium and that it had produced the particular substance that was an active anti-parasitic agent. Fermentation chemists and biologists at Merck isolated this substance and managed to get the bacterium to make even more of it. Analytical chemists figured out its chemical structure.

We called it 'avermectin'. The name was a nod to the drug's biological action. So often, drugs are named according to their chemical attributes, and I wanted to plant a flag, so to speak, for biology. So I made up a mongrel word to be distinctive and that incorporated the drug's biological attributes: the 'a' refers to 'not', the 'verm' draws on the Latin for worm, and the 'ectin' refers to ectoparasites, because ivermectin is active against external parasites, such as lice and mites, as well as parasitic worms.

Then, synthetic chemists and parasitologists worked together to alter the chemical structure to make it even more effective against parasites. I have huge respect and admiration for everyone involved in that process. My friends in chemistry concede that a microbe can make a substance that a human chemist could never dream of making, but they take the attitude that only chemists can make it right! And that is what they did. They made thousands of derivatives (versions of the chemical the bacterium had produced) in a bid to make versions that could work even more effectively. They sent us the derivatives and we tested them out against parasites.

The result of this process was a molecule with a chemical structure that was similar to that of avermectin but with added hydrogens. At first it was thought the most suitable name for such a thing might be 'hyvermectin', until it was pointed out that in some languages the word 'hyver' means testicle. Change of plan: it was named ivermectin!

In tests, ivermectin proved a potent agent that could kill a wide range of parasitic worms found in the internal organs of mammals, as well as killing many disease-causing insects, but it was a little more nuanced than that. For one thing, when I say 'killing' I am referring to the worms being paralysed, and then the body disposing of them. Parasites can be a particularly complicated target for drug treatment, because they go through different stages in their life cycles, and a potential drug might be good at stopping the parasite at one stage of its life cycle but not at another stage.

My own research on dog heartworm disease offers a case in point. When a dog becomes infected with heartworm (*Dirofilaria immitis*), the worms establish themselves in the animal and go through their life cycle of young worms maturing into the adult form. The adult worms can make dogs extremely ill, and can even kill them, so it's an important parasite to control. But if you kill the adult worm while it is in the dog, the result can be catastrophic for the dog, because the dead adult worms can collect in the lung. In the lab, Lyndia Blair and I discovered that ivermectin could kill both the first and second developmental stages of heartworm in dogs—but not the more mature, older stages.

This meant that ivermectin could wipe out larvae that had entered a dog anytime during the month following treatment— not because the drug remains in the body but because ivermectin kills those two successive developmental stages of the parasite. That gave ivermectin a very big advantage over other drugs. It now became possible to develop a commercial product that needs to be given only once a month instead of daily (as was the case with older anti-heartworm medications).

Now there are more drugs on the market to treat this parasite, but if you have ever wondered why vets advise you to give your dog a regular dose of worming tablets, this is one of the reasons—it's to kill off the young larvae and nip any infection in the bud. Our heartworm programme at Merck was remarkably successful, and ivermectin was brought to the market as a preventative medicine for the disease in dogs

Ivermectin had indeed cleared all the hurdles impressively. It was effective at low doses, it was well tolerated (which means it had few side-effects), it could be given by mouth or injection, it was chemically stable so it didn't need to be refrigerated or have any other privileged treatment, and of course it worked against a range of parasites, including some that had become resistant to other drugs. Ivermectin went on the market in 1981 under various brand names for different applications, and just three years later it was the world's top animal pharmaceutical. In all that time, there was, to my knowledge, no communal eureka moment. It just didn't happen. Things were all starting to fit together but we were just working away and still thinking of what experiment we were going to do tomorrow, so maybe in some ways it seems strange but there was no particular moment of shared celebration across the many groups that contributed, it all just progressed.

For me the wonderful thing about this process of going from a soil sample to a chemical agent that can reduce the burden of disease, is that while it was an incredibly complex and technically difficult endeavour, it originated in a very simple experiment. Complexity was built on simplicity. That is a critical lesson. We fed that mouse an unknown amount of an unknown substance that might not be there, and we watched what happened. From that experiment we found the key to what became a blockbuster anti-parasitic drug.

Joining the dots:
from heartworm to river blindness

It sounds like a big leap: to take a drug that treats heartworm in dogs and use it to treat river blindness in humans. It was a jump alright, but it wasn't done in one giant leap. It was a series of insights and hunches that slowly but surely joined the dots and, just as in the discovery of ivermectin itself, it involved many people with different backgrounds and a deep understanding of basic biology.

We were working on the development of ivermectin, and Lyndia Blair, by now a senior parasitologist and technician in my lab at Merck, read a paper about how horses are commonly infected with a parasitic worm called *Onchocerca*. This was a real find. The parasite didn't cause disease in horses, it was a bit of a zoological oddity, and that meant veterinarians were not really aware of it.

My colleague John Egerton was carrying out other tests on horses, and because of this new information, he carried out additional tests to see if ivermectin might have an effect on infections of *Onchocerca*. Those tests showed that the drug killed the larvae (that is, the progeny) of the worms. John reported the data to me in a typically matter-of-fact memo. This finding prompted me to wonder if ivermectin might work against another species of *Onchocerca* worm, *Onchocerca volvulus*, the one that causes river blindness in humans.

This was an important question to ask. While I worked predominantly on medicines for veterinary use, I always had an active interest in human parasitology. As mentioned previously, I had worked on the schistosome program in Merck, which looked at the parasitic agent responsible for snail fever, a major human disease. More significantly, my involvement in the New York Society of Tropical Medicine, and my annual teaching duties at New York College of Medicine, had made me very aware of the big, and all too often neglected, problem of parasitic diseases in humans. Not surprisingly, given my line of work, I was especially aware of what treatments were, or were not, available for the various tropical diseases. River blindness is a truly devastating disease. Humans become exposed to it when they are bitten by a blackfly carrying the *Onchocerca volvulus* parasite—the fly breeds in rivers in some tropical regions. The *Onchocerca volvulus* worm enters the bite site and establishes an infection in the human. The adult worms produce larvae, or microfilariae, and these travel to the skin and the eye where they cause itching and inflammation. The itch is extremely intense, and in severe infections, the skin becomes damaged and scarred. Worst of all, the body's immune system can react to the infection in a way that causes the front of the eye to become opaque, leading to the loss of sight. Existing treatments for the disease were far from satisfactory.

In 1977 I wrote a memo to my boss in Merck, Jerry Birnbaum, telling him that we had seen that ivermectin was effective against *Onchocerca* in horses. I explained the link to river blindness and pointed out that ivermectin could be transformative here. I proposed that we look at *Onchocerca* in other animal species next. He was impressed and I got funding for another trial, this time working with Bruce Copeman in Townsville University in Queensland, Australia. I had come to know Bruce and learned about his work on cattle when I met him at a parasitology conference in Europe—the advantage to going to conferences is that it broadens your horizons and expands your contact book—and we set up a trial to see if ivermectin could affect a type of *Onchocerca* that was found in cattle. It did, and again it killed the young larvae of the parasite.

So now we knew that ivermectin could tackle larvae of related *Onchocerca* worms in cattle and horses. The question then was this: would it work specifically against the larval progeny of *Onchocerca volvulus*, the parasite that was causing such untold human suffering, loss of independence and ability to work for millions of people in affected regions of the world?

In 1978 I wrote another memo to Jerry Birnbaum, highlighting how exciting it was that ivermectin could kill the larval progeny of *Onchocerca* in cattle and horses. It was particularly exciting because of the key role played by the larval progeny of *Onchocerca volvulus* in the skin damage and eye damage associated with river blindness. Our new findings suggested that ivermectin's action against that particular life-cycle stage could well be effective in alleviating the signs and symptoms of river blindness. Further, if treated people no longer had the parasites in their skin, then the blackflies would no longer pick up the parasites and transmit them to other people. In other words, there was even the possibility of stopping the transmission of river blindness in a region. I suggested talking to the World Health Organization about the best course of action from the medical, political and commercial points of view.

Dr Birnbaum immediately grasped the significance of this suggestion, and this memo got fed further up the chain. A little later, Roy Vagelos, who was the head of Merck Research, wrote a personal note to me (copy to Birnbaum) strongly endorsing further research into the potential human applications.

Around the same time, I wrote to the World Health Organization to engage them in discussions, and I prepared background information for Merck clinical personnel who were to discuss the testing of avermectins (including ivermectin) against human diseases. In 1980 the toss of a coin decided that one of Merck's medical directors, Mohammed Aziz, would oversee the trial of ivermectin in humans to treat river blindness. Dr Aziz had been raised and medically trained in Bangladesh and he had worked with the World Health Organization in tropical Africa. He was a deeply caring physician and ideally suited to this task.

The coin toss came about because Merck was planning trials on two different drug candidates—ivermectin for river blindness and another compound against the parasite that causes Chagas disease. Kenneth Brown and Dr Aziz were each to lead one, and the coin decreed that Dr Aziz lead the river blindness trial, though he worked closely with Dr Brown on it.

After much planning, the first river blindness trial took place in Dakar, Senegal, in 1981. Thirty-two men who were infected with the *Onchocerca volvulus* parasite took part: some received ivermectin and others received a placebo. Six weeks later, the ones who had received the ivermectin had a greatly reduced parasite burden in their skin, and in some cases the parasites had been eliminated. This was encouraging and it pointed the way to larger trials. There were still lots of hurdles to clear before ivermectin could be an effective treatment for the millions of people who needed it, but we were heading in the right direction.

Onchocerca

Onchocerca volvulus is a parasitic worm. Its microscopic larval stage is responsible for river blindness and skin disease in humans. The skin disease is caused by migration of numerous microscopic larvae through the skin of infected people—a migration that is essential for the completion of the parasite life cycle. Invasion of the eye by the parasites is not needed for parasite propagation, but eye damage and blindness occur when the parasites happen to penetrate the eye after migrating through the nearby skin. I reflected on this in a poem.

Onchocerca

I don't need your goddam eye!

All I need is a bit of skin
big enough to me to scatter
a few larvae in,

just enough to make it probable
that there'll be a pick-up
and delivery.

Don't look at me that way—
I don't need your goddam eye.

The donation that changed millions of lives

Scientific research does not exist in a vacuum. It is a human activity and in many cases it can have an impact on humans and on society at large. In the case of ivermectin, the science was solid. But it would have no impact on river blindness unless the drug was available and accessible to the people who needed it, and most of the people who needed it could not afford to buy medicines. That's why Merck's decision to make ivermectin freely available for use in the treatment of river blindness was so important.

The donation arose from a dilemma within Merck, more specifically within its Corporate Human Health marketing division. In 1986 that group, including Robert Fluss, Thomas Casola and Charles Fettig, had two objectives; first priority: make ivermectin available to the vast numbers of people suffering from river blindness; second priority: generate a financial return on investment. The objectives being clearly irreconcilable, the group concluded that the only solution was donation of the drug. Obviously, that would have to be approved by top management. In reaching a decision to approve such an extraordinary measure, Merck's then CEO, Roy Vagelos, had input from close associates. One of them was Edward Scolnick who had succeeded Vagelos as president of the Merck Research laboratories, and he is on record as having been in favour of donation. Others may have supported it too. Nevertheless, accountability for the decision was held by Dr Vagelos alone, and he approved the donation. In fact, as he later recalled, he had not alerted the Merck board of directors about it by the time the donation was announced, but later had assurance that they would have supported the move had they been asked beforehand.

It was the right thing to do. It would be, for many reasons, a difficult thing to do. And it would be expensive. For one thing, Merck would have to invest in the trials and development of this drug for humans—one couldn't just take the ivermectin as developed for use in cattle or dogs and adjust the dose. The regulatory process rightly required a separate schedule of trials and monitoring. The immediate problem, however, was How could it be done?

Senior Merck executives John Lyons and Jerry Jackson went to the Carter Center in Georgia and consulted Bill Foege, head of the Task Force for Child Survival. He had played a major role in the smallpox eradication campaign and had served as head of the Centers for Disease Control and Prevention before joining former US president Jimmy Carter's medical programme. The Merck emissaries must have been persuasive in describing the company's commitment to the donation of ivermectin for use against river blindness, because Foege and his associates agreed to work up a practicable plan. The result was a corporate–public partnership that was a marvellous breakthrough in itself. It had a close liaison with the Onchocerciasis Control Programme and was built on two initiatives. The first was the formation of a Mectizan Expert Committee (the human formulation of iver-mectin is named Mectizan), consisting of tropical medicine experts from a variety of international institutions. Foege himself was persuaded to head it (another breakthrough!). Merck would be represented only by a non-voting member. The second initia-tive was the creation of a Mectizan Donation Programme, as the implementation arm of the endeavour. Applications and proto-cols for participation in the distribution and delivery of medicine would be approved by the expert committee and carried out by the donation programme. As well as providing cost-free ivermec-tin, Merck would pay for the cost of getting the medicine to the border of the country in which it would be used, as well as the appliable customs fees and such.

From the outset, the operation expanded to become a vast coa-lition of agencies. In addition to the World Health Organization and the World Bank there were numerous governmental and non-governmental aid organisations, charitable medical organ-isations and others. It was fortunate that Robert S. McNamara, president of the World Bank, had given the bank an entirely new focus on the welfare of people in the developing regions of the world, and that McNamara himself took a strong interest in the alleviation of river blindness. Under the leadership of Bruce

Benton, the World Bank funded grants that enabled much of the work that was done in this complex, yet effective, push toward the control of the disease.

In 1987 I travelled with Dr Vagelos and Dr Birnbaum in a small plane to Washington, D.C., for the announcement that ivermectin was to be donated for use in treating river blindness. This was a high-profile event, including a speech from Senator Edward Kennedy. The atmosphere was one of hope and celebration, and the news was greeted favourably. Cynics may have suspected that the donation was a PR stunt or some kind of tax break for the company, but I think it was done because it was morally the right thing to do. The creation of the Mectizan Expert Committee and the Mectizan Donation Program triggered a massive outpouring of support from numerous aid agencies around the world. Their combined efforts made it possible to achieve the very complex management of the ivermectin donation programme and the very difficult on-the-ground delivery of the drug to patients in countries affected by river blindness—often in resource-poor or conflict-stricken parts of the world. The success that followed undoubtedly owes much to Foege's vision and his belief in the effectiveness of close coalitions of persons and parties driven by passionate commitment to human welfare and unhampered by excessive concern for administrative lines and divisions. Among those parties were, in addition to the World Bank, the World Health Organization, Helen Keller International, Sightsavers, the Carter Foundation and others.

The Carter Foundation is a humanitarian organisation set up by the former president. I met him a couple of times in connection with his river blindness work, but Mary and I had met his wife, Rosalynn, before that. When Jimmy Carter ran for the presidency in the mid-1970s, his wife campaigned for him. Friends of ours in New Jersey hosted a reception in their home where Mrs Carter spoke. In chatting with her at that event, I was impressed by her eager and expert defense of her husband's policies. President Carter always seemed to be natural and at ease, and he has been indefatigable in his support of the Mectizan Donation Program.

More than 30 years later, and taking into account the distribution of ivermectin for the prevention of filariasis (elephantiasis) and other diseases, more than three billion ivermectin treatments have been donated. River blindness has been certified as eradicated in almost all endemic regions of South and Central America. In sub-Saharan Africa, the burden of suffering blindness has been vastly reduced for millions of people, and in some regions the transmission cycle of the parasite has been halted.

I often hear expressions of amazement about the sheer magnitude of this undertaking, and indeed I share that feeling. It has been, and continues to be, an undertaking of colossal commitment in areas of science, corporate responsibility, public-health management, international and inter-agency cooperation, communication and good will. It was built on the heroic tropical field-work of those who established the human safety and effectiveness of the drug. It was an undertaking that led to a transformation in individual lives. It was the right thing to do. And for me there is also another, more primal, impression. I am awestruck by the transmutation of a substance. It was stuff in a laboratory bottle. And it was made into a medicine—a medicine that brought and continues to bring enormous relief from human suffering.

Compassion and research

In 2012 I reflected on compassion in research in an email to David Addiss, the then director of Children Without Worms, an organisation committed to the global control of intestinal worm infections:

> Compassion! I am not sure I share your hope that compassion was a pervasive factor in the development of Mectizan, and so am inclined to agree that we should hesitate to claim it.
>
> Any researcher with a shred of decency is going to rejoice when research findings turn out to be of benefit to humans either directly (as, for example, in controlling human disease) or indirectly (as, for example, in increasing the production of the food and fiber needed—or at least demanded—by most human populations). But it would be a rare researcher who could justly claim that compassion had been the prime motivation for doing the research.
>
> I take it as a given that many, perhaps most, physicians can justly claim that compassion was a significant motivation for their entering the medical profession. You [as a physician] would be in a better position than I am to judge the degree to which compassion motivates non-clinical research done by a physician. I expect it depends on the specific circumstances.
>
> None of this, of course, has anything to do with whether physicians or non-physicians (or liberals or conservatives, or artists or engineers, or inhabitants of East or of West) are more or less compassionate as people. The decision to donate Mectizan, and the implementation of the donation, involved non-scientists as well as

scientists—and probably involved a mixture of motivations. I am not among the cynics who point to such legitimate, but non-heroic, motives as tax-write-offs. (The actual tax benefits in this case are, I am told, negligible.)

Nor do I buy the suggestion that the donation decision was made to boost the morale of Merck employees. If Merck employees thought that corporate management had made the decision to boost employee morale, employee morale would not have been boosted. Having been one of them, I believe that Merck employees felt proud because they believed the Company had done the right thing; and furthermore they believed that the Company had done the right thing because it was the right thing.

Compassion, I like to think, was not absent from the Mectizan enterprise; but I suspect that its role as motivator can never be known. There can be, I think, a sense of rectitude within a corporation, and that, too, may have played a part.

Three years after that letter was written, the role of compassion was raised in a panel discussion during Nobel Week in Stockholm. 'Nobel Minds' is a television program produced jointly by Swedish Television and the BBC, and hosted by Zainab Badawi. As a member of the 'Nobel Minds' discussion panel of 2015, I was asked whether my work on the control of parasitic disease had been motivated by compassion. I said that it had not. As the discussion continued, I was gratified to find that not a single member of the panel laid claim to compassion as a primary motivator of their Nobel-winning work.

Tension under the big tree—
treating river blindness

One of the most emotionally rewarding and personally fulfilling episodes of my involvement with ivermectin was travelling to Togo and Burkina-Faso in West Africa in the late 1980s to observe the Mectizan programmes in action there. The medicine, at that time, had been approved for human use, people were taking it in sub-Saharan Africa and its effects were being evaluated and monitored at the community level.

One of the stand-out moments took place under a great big tree; not immensely tall, but with limbs extending luxuriously in all directions, casting a huge circle of welcome shade on the sandy soil. Gathered in that shade were a few dozen Africans and three (conspicuously white) Westerners, myself among them.

A few of the Africans were seated in deck chairs. Some were village elders, and one was a young doctor from Mali, Mamadou Bah, who worked for the Onchocerciasis (River Blindness) Control Program. He had been assigned to administer the Mectizan treatment programme in this remote part of Togo. Also in deck chairs were the three travellers—Bruce Dull, Stuart Kingma and myself. Standing in the big semi-circle was the entire population of two villages. The scene was reminiscent of a very old movie. The atmosphere was tense, but I did not find it alarming.

One set of villagers lived there, in the village with the big tree. They had gathered at the tree, by prior arrangement, to receive their Mectizan pills. The visiting population from another village had arrived, with no prior arrangement, for the same purpose. But there was a problem: in those early days of Mectizan distribution, a village could not be treated at a moment's notice. That needed planning, demographic documentation, the mobilisation of resources, money for transportation and so on.

The villagers who had arrived unannounced at this place had missed an earlier round of Mectizan treatment, because their village was too isolated. They built a road to provide access to their village, but somehow they had again been missed. This time, hearing of an impending visit by a Mectizan team to another village in their region, they had marched over a mountain in the night, and now here they were, calmly presenting themselves for treatment along with the local inhabitants.

What they received instead was the news that treatment was precluded by the lack of preparation and logistical support. This led to the chiefs of both villages engaging in intense discussion under the big tree. We foreigners could not understand the language they used, but Dr Bah explained the situation.

At length, it was agreed that the resident population would receive its Mectizan treatment and that the visiting villagers would receive their treatment another day soon. The crowd dispersed, but all was not well. An extension of this mission would need fuel for vehicles and lodgings for medical and support staff, costing money, but no additional expenditure had been authorised. Later that day, in the nearest town, the young doctor sent a telex to headquarters, asking for authorisation to carry out Mectizan treatment in the second village. He added that the money for the extension of the project could be taken out of his salary, if necessary.

Happily, it was not necessary! But that offer, made so matter-of-factly, is not something I will forget. Many other vivid memories of Africa have also stayed with me. The savannah villages were quite different from New Jersey towns. Seeing people with river blindness was different from reading about them. The little, white Mectizan pill seemed very different from the crude material we had worked with in the laboratory. It was all different, it was all fascinating. But what I remember most vividly was that afternoon under the big tree.

Efforts had been afoot for several years to reduce the populations of blackflies that carry the *Onchocerca* parasite, to try to disrupt the cycle of transmission. This was carried out by the Onchocerca Control Program, supported by the World Health Organization with the World Bank and other agencies. This particular initiative involved putting insecticides in rivers and other bodies of water. It was complicated and expensive to administer, needed to be monitored for ecological damage, and needed the co-operation of agencies and communities. Nevertheless, it was brilliantly executed and very effective. The advent of ivermectin and the Mectizan Donation Program changed the thrust of the international campaign to control river blindness. It was as an observer of that pharmaceutical approach that I had come to Africa.

During that work, I had the privilege of meeting chiefs of many villages, who often led by example for their people by being the first to take ivermectin. They were, without exception, marvellously impressive. They had an aura of authority about them, and with the help of translators were easy to talk to. One of the chiefs asked me about my work, and we talked about it. Then, with a big smile, he joked that I should 'find the cause of death and lock it in a box'.

One of the outstanding leaders of the campaign to control river blindness was Ibrahim Samba, who hailed from The Gambia and had studied medicine at University College Dublin and completed his training in surgery at Edinburgh. I recall being with him in a restaurant that was run by local nuns. As well as menus, they had hymn sheets, and when the time came to sing, Dr Samba sang heartily. He certainly got into the spirit of it.

I had gone to West Africa to see ivermectin being administered in several remote communities. I was driven around in a vehicle with ONCHO written on its side—one trip involved a nine-hour journey from Burkina-Faso to Togo. There were helicopters and fixed-wing planes bearing those letters too. As a parasitologist, I thought it was quite something to see the nickname of a parasite thus emblazoned on high-tech equipment. On that visit to observe the Mectizan programme it was just wonderful to see the culmination of the research we had done. What had started with a microbe and a mouse was now a medicine to help humans, to alleviate suffering. That experience will always stay with me.

A short note on drug discovery

There are many ways to find a new drug. One can set one's sights on a particular biochemical pathway or process in the body, then home in on that target. This is the 'rational' approach. Or one can cast the net wide and screen potential sources of drugs, observing their effects until something clicks.

The latter is the empirical approach, and it is one I have favoured in practice throughout my career. Taking the empirical approach led us to drugs that have made a real difference, including ivermectin, thiabendazole, pyrantel and levamisole. Yet, as new techniques in biology emerged in the late twentieth century—and particularly techniques in molecular biology—the trend moved away from empirical research. It was seen as 'old hat'. This was, I believe, to the detriment of my career personally, and (far more important) I believe it has been to the detriment of global health.

We need new drugs to treat infectious diseases more effectively, and we urgently need new drugs to address the problem of resistance to existing drugs. To do this, I believe we should keep looking for them (the empirical approach) as well as designing them (the rational approach). Looking for them with the empirical approach involves trial and error, astute observation and 'random' (mechanism-blind) screening for activity. Some find the concept of such work intellectually humiliating, an attitude that is philosophically insupportable.

There is nothing irrational about the use of empiricism in scientific research. It is a lesson, however, that seems to be resisted by, or simply neglected by, a surprisingly large number of people: over the centuries, much progress in science has come from empirical sources—that is, from the exploitation of chance event, observation, or trial-and-error investigation. The drugs used to treat bacterial or parasitic diseases have virtually all come to us through development of empirical findings. If we ignore that history, we will fail to repeat it. That will be a self-inflicted tragedy (though we will not know about it).

I am not in any way disparaging the rational approach—it has yielded important medicines in areas other than that of infectious diseases. But it has long seemed to me that in the pursuit of new drugs, many pursuers fail to recognise the particular pitfall of viewing the empirical approach as intrinsically inferior to the rational. We belittle and ignore the empirical approach at our peril. We will never know how many precious drugs we might have discovered had we not failed to apply common sense.

I have urged that we undertake a more thorough scouring of Earth in all its ecological niches for organisms of all kinds that might produce unusual and interesting biochemicals. Such activity is underway in many parts of the world, but we need a more concerted effort. This would require organisation, collaboration and motivation, but the harvest could be fruitful for the future of humanity.

One of the joys of my early years of work on therapeutic agents was the realisation that every new drug is a new tool, not only for study of the drug and its applications, but for studies in basic science as well. As a general principle, any novel pharmacological agent should be tested, as soon as it becomes available, in almost any laboratory assay. Such work should be done with the expectation of failure but the possibility of success (keeping in mind that the perceived value of success should far outweigh the cost of failure).

From murderer to scientist

Nathan Leopold was the most notorious murderer I ever met. Actually, he is the only murderer I ever met (well ... so far as I know). In 1924 Leopold and another young man, Richard Loeb, killed a young boy. They were caught, and after a sensational and famous trial, they were sentenced to spend the rest of their lives in Illinois State Prison. There, Loeb was himself murdered, and we are left with Leopold.

In prison, Leopold was a compulsive learner. He became an x-ray technician in the prison hospital; he ran a correspondence school; read widely and became very knowledgeable on such subjects as philosophy, statistics and theology. Not surprisingly, when a malaria research program was started at the hospital, he became deeply involved. He devised an improved method of counting parasites in blood smears—though I cannot vouch for his claims—and he gave tutorials and laboratory demonstrations to the other prisoners.

In the mid-twentieth century, Leopold volunteered to take part in experiments that helped in the search for anti-malarial drugs. The routine was for the volunteer to be bitten by ten mosquitoes carrying the malaria parasite, *Plasmodium vivax*. Leopold came down with a severe case of malaria, but survived. He was treated with two different experimental drugs that paved the way for the drug Primaquine, which made radical cure of malaria feasible for the first time, and the drug became enormously important for that reason.

In 1957, because of a legal technicality and because he was one of those who 'had voluntarily risked their lives' for the health of the armed forces, Leopold was released on parole—and after 33 years in jail, he moved to Puerto Rico to live out the remaining years of his life. He did some research for the Puerto Rican Department of Health, and it was that research that led to my meeting with him. The department was concerned about the prevalence of intestinal worms in the children of the rural poor. It was known that intestinal nematode worms are spread among people via faeces, and Leopold and his colleague Howard Stanton wondered if there might be contamination within households and in the damp sandy yards where the children played.

The contamination would not be obvious, but Leopold had an idea—he thought he would arrange for a group of children to swallow fluorescent paint! This would pass through the intestines and out in the faeces, and even tiny amounts of fecal material would then be detectable with the aid of an ultra-violet lamp. It is not quite as outrageous as it might seem at first. The pigment would not be expected to be absorbed from the gut, and besides, Leopold had toxicology data on it. Leopold, Stanton and another colleague even did a human safety trial: they each swallowed some of the stuff and they all felt fine! They knew that their safety assessment was far from ideal, but it was the best they could do. So they gave doses of the pigment to 54 people who were otherwise going about their ordinary family activities in their homes; and after a strategic wait, they went around with their UV lamp. The method worked! They detected fluorescence—indirect evidence of fecal contamination—in many places in and around the home: on the surface of furniture, on toys and on people's hands.

Leopold never finished the work, and never published it. He was quite ill by this time, and died in the following year, but before that happened I had the opportunity to discuss the project with him. I was interested, having myself learned the techniques of fecal examination by hunting for worm eggs in the feces of children in Puerto Rico's rural slums.

Leopold was portly and avuncular. When we met, he was impeccably dressed in a dark business suit. He was articulate and knowledgeable, and he was exuberant about his current research. His command of the technical language was assured. It struck me as an odd juxtaposition: Leopold the murderer took opportunities to become involved in medical parasitology and in research aimed at benefiting humankind, yet hovering over our chat was the spectre of grisly murder, the ghost of Leopold the killer—unacknowledged, of course, by either of us.

That lack of acknowledgement now reminds me of a much more ordinary chat I once had with Horace Stunkard, who at the time was one of the greatest parasitologists alive. I had come to know him through the New York Society of Tropical Medicine, and we found ourselves sitting together at a big banquet during a joint meeting of the British and American societies of tropical medicine. As Stunkard was cutting his steak, a sizable chunk of meat skidded off his knife and jumped right over to my plate. I was somewhat in awe of him, of course, and was hoping that he hadn't noticed where it had landed; and he, I suppose, was hoping that I hadn't seen it arriving. In any case we carried right on without acknowledging that anything had happened.

In the same vein, when I was chatting with Leopold in a conference lounge, I knew that he was that Leopold, but I don't know if he knew that I knew that he was that Leopold. I was careful not to ask him about his past. He didn't ask me about my past, either; but, then, my past was a good deal less 'colourful' than his.

Leopold developed a plan to conduct a more meaningful study of the safety of his pigment in humans. He recruited the necessary volunteers among prisoners in the nearby state penitentiary. But the ethical acceptability of using prison volunteers had been overturned in the years since Leopold himself had served in that role. He owed his parole to his volunteer service, but was denied permission to use prison volunteers for his proposed safety assessment. I have no doubt that he, being something of a philosopher, understood and accepted the situation.

Life after Merck. Retirement? What retirement?

In 1990, after 33 years working at Merck, I retired. The company hosted a lavish retirement dinner for me, at which colleagues gathered and people gave speeches. Mary and Betsy were there, and the whole event was very special and fulfilling. Looking back, I think I could say the same about my time at Merck—it was very special and fulfilling. There had been some rough spots. Throughout my tenure, however, I admired the company and the ethos on which it had been built. I admired the talents of its people. The arc of my career had been marked by the introduction of thiabendazole (the first of the anti-nematode benzimidazoles) at its beginning; marked by the introduction of rafoxanide emerging from my liver-fluke foray in the middle; and marked by the pharmacological breakthrough of ivermectin at the end. These, as well as cambendazole, clorsulon and eprinomectin at various career points, were all products of our empirical screening, and all were discovered in a setting of exhilarating science, constant publishing and active involvement in professional societies. Looking back at my career in industry and in academia, it seems impossible to imagine how anyone could have been more fortunate in their pursuit of a livelihood.

Over the decades of which I speak, a seismic shift had occurred in the world of biology. The molecular biology revolution has affected the many branches of science, including mine. Molecules are no longer mere clusters of atoms. They are infinitely complex, and they include the nucleic acids that control life at the most basic level. They are, consequently, central to scientific research—not only in academia but in the pharmaceutical industry. Molecular biology would now be called upon for the discovery of new antiparasitic drugs. As the twentieth century neared its end, an era that had brought Merck great prosperity through its antiparasitic products was also drawing to a close.

I had been director of Merck's department of parasitology over a period of eighteen years (six of them as senior director), with a four-year interruption for service as director of the company's Veterinary Research and Development Laboratory in Australia, and subsequent administrative adjustments. In 1984 the department of parasitology was put under the leadership of scientists committed to the 'rational approach'—to the goal of devising, rather than finding, molecules exhibiting efficacy against bacterial and parasitic infections. I was relieved of the title of 'Director of Parasitology', and in 1988 my area of responsibility was further constricted. I continued my research; the ivermectin programme seeming to offer endless opportunities for experimentation. Still, being a veteran of an earlier era in biology, approaching the age of 60 years, and no longer holding the position to which I had become accustomed, I was open to the lure of retirement and the possibilities that retirement could offer. And, right on cue, a great possibility came along! Merck offered an enhanced retirement 'package' to employees who were ready for early retirement and were also ready to make a commitment to teach mathematics or science for a certain period. University teaching had always appealed to me and I had been doing some all along. Thus, the time was right to move on, and I did. I started a new position the day after my retirement. Mary says jokingly that she never had to worry about me getting in the way, a retiree kicking around the house!

Drew University is a private university in Madison, New Jersey, and has a remarkable, indeed unique, programme called the Research Institute for Scientists Emeriti—RISE. It exists to enable retired experts from industry to remain active in their research fields while supervising the research of undergraduate students. Shortly before my retirement, I was invited to give a lecture at Drew University's department of biology. The head of biology asked me if I had heard of the Scientists Emeriti program, which I had. He suggested I go upstairs and talk to its director, George deStevens, which I did. So I became a RISE Fellow and, over the next 20 years, I had the enjoyment of mentoring and supervising several motivated, bright and hard-working undergraduate students in their research projects at Drew. Mentoring in the field of parasitology was exactly what I wanted to do.

When I started, my new lab was starkly empty. The cleaners had been thorough—there were empty cabinets, empty shelves, empty drawers; not even a test tube or Petri dish in sight. Yet there, in one cabinet, was a single object, an unopened bottle of chloroform. (I did not view it as a sinister message.) The cleaners had clearly known about strictures on disposal of 'hazardous materials' and so I had inherited an abandoned item of hazardous material.

Worms are never far from my thoughts. That was true even when pondering one of my other favourite subjects, the history of medicine. In the history of anaesthesia, ether was followed by chloroform as an agent for putting people to sleep during surgery. I began to wonder if chloroform could put a worm to sleep. The lab was quickly fitted out with glassware, plasticware, microscopes and other accoutrements of a biology lab. A very special new addition was a culture of the tiny (almost microscopic) free-living nematode worm *Caenorhabditis elegans*. Naturally, I put some of the worms in a dish of saline, added a drop of dilute chloroform, and watched them under a dissecting microscope to see what would happen. The worms stopped moving. When I removed the chloroform by means of a series of saline rinses, the worms started moving again. I could not claim that the worms had gone to sleep; but they had certainly undergone a reversible suspension of normal motility.

Then the very bright undergraduate student Heidi Smith arrived into the lab. We set to work to capitalise on the potential rewards of having found a bottle of chloroform. After I had set up an initial experiment for Heidi, she came to my office and tentatively suggested that I had made a mistake with a decimal point in one of the dilutions. I thought this was wonderful! Some might have just used the wrong solution in the experiment without noticing. Others might have noticed but not have told me. But she had the confidence to notice and to tell me.

Together, we demonstrated that ivermectin could paralyse *C. elegans* worms not only under normal circumstances, but also when the worms were in an alcoholic stupor and incapable of ingesting the drug. This was not a trivial exercise. We were trying to shed light on an unresolved question: does a nematode worm become paralysed as a result of ingesting ivermectin; or does the drug instead (or also) enter the worm through the surface or through other orifices? Our results supported the latter option.

When we submitted a report of our findings to a refereed journal, I was eager to hear back from the editor. When the unmistakable journal envelope arrived, I opened it with more suspense and excitement than had been the case with many of my own publications. The paper was accepted and published, and Heidi's career as a biomedical researcher was off to a good start.

Despite their busy schedules, several other students in my lab also published papers on the research we did together, and that was exceptionally rewarding. One student, Miten Patel, manged to spend a lot of time in my lab, and actually published three papers by the time he graduated. One day, he said he wanted to try out a talk he was hoping to present at a local science conference. Then, on the spot, he proceeded to give me the entire talk, solicited my comments, and went on to win a prestigious first prize at the conference. Not surprisingly, he has been very successful in his career as a medical oncologist.

In mentoring students, I found it useful to start off by setting up an experiment or two for them, so that it was fairly easy for them to carry out the experiments while at the same time becoming familiar with the equipment and procedures of the lab. Soon, we would begin to talk about options for different experiments and I would encourage the students to develop their own ideas and follow their curiosity, removing the 'scaffolding' as their confidence and skills grew. It was important to view the partnership as two minds focused on the same question, working together. It was a privilege just to be there as these young people discovered the difference between a classroom exercise and actual research—when they realise that they are doing an experiment that has never been done before, so they are finding out something previously unknown. That is a time of ongoing magic, and it is, I think, when researchers are born.

One of the things I also tried to instil in their minds is the desirability of doing research as soon as possible when they finish their undergraduate degrees and go on to graduate school. Initially of course they would need to work with a professor or another experienced mentor who could guide them, but after a while they could come up with their own ideas for new questions to ask, or new experiments to do. I encouraged them, when they got to that stage, to talk to their professors and to ask if they could try things out. By getting some ownership in the ongoing research, they would be able to build aptitude for research, and that would carry over into the next phases of their careers. For me, mentoring students was a great privilege and I did it, unsalaried, for the love of it, for twenty years. It was where I wanted to be.

An unexpected honour from the
US National Academy of Sciences

My election to the National Academy of Sciences should have made me more prepared for the emotional impact that would follow the announcement of the Nobel prize. For quite a while, I was unaware that I had been nominated for membership of the National Academy of Sciences, and when the results of the 2001 elections were announced in the newspapers, I went into a 'tailspin' of worry as to whether I was qualified to receive that honour.

It turned out that my nominators had been Boyd Woodruff, a former student of Nobel laureate Selman Waxman and, like me, a retiree from the Merck laboratories, and Arnold Demain, a long-time professor of microbiology at Massachusetts Institute of Technology. Dr Woodruff later recalled that he talked to me, one-to-one, for an hour-and-a-half while he persuaded me not to decline my membership in the National Academy (he divulged that it had received a rare 100% vote from the relevant committee). My election was by then a *fait accompli,* and I decided that I should not try to repudiate it.

Still, I was extremely uncomfortable because of my awareness that I had been just one member of a large team in the development of Merck's arsenal of antiparasitic drugs. I had gone so far as to publish a letter to the editor, calling attention to the central importance of teamwork in the case of ivermectin. Now, I have come to the conclusion that if you have respect for your profession (and if you don't, you might consider looking for a different one) then you should be candid and forthrightly insistent regarding credit for priority in discovery. Socially, if you have respect and affection for your family and friends (and if you don't, the problem cannot be addressed here) you should be candid and accurate about credit, but yet tolerant of the excesses that come your way from kind hearts. Your friends, after all, don't give a hoot for your unseen team-mates.

Socially, the positive side of this whole National Academy thing was the installation ceremony in Washington, D.C. Family and friends were invited to enjoy concerts, receptions, excursions and banquets, as well as scientific symposia. A solemn moment was the signing of a big book of member signatures. There are now several volumes of signatures, but it continues the series begun by order of President Abraham Lincoln when he founded the academy in the mid-nineteenth century. A far-from-solemn, and indeed delightfully light-hearted, occasion was the opportunity to visit, climb on and sit on, the huge bronze statue of Einstein placed outdoors on the academy grounds.

Microscopes: looking through and at them

My interest in microscopes began, as interests often do, without intent or premonitory symptoms; and it all began with one pathetic little microscope. It was by no means a Trinity College instrument, but within the Trinity community it was casually handed off to anyone who thought they could make some passing use of it when cramming for a practical exam.

I found, as others had found, that it was cumbersome to use in comparison to the college microscopes. It was, after all, about 100 years old—not that anyone thought of it as an antique! It was considered so worthless and outdated that money was never involved in its haphazard passage from person to person. I suspect that it had been bought at Dublin's Moore Street market, which in those days had lots of bric-a-brac, and was a place where students could browse for kitchen gadgets and curios for their rooms in college. I took the microscope to Ramelton to prepare for an exam (held at the end of vacation, not at the end of term). I am not sure if I used it, but when a cousin asked to borrow it, I readily passed it on.

Two-dozen years later I saw a somewhat similar microscope in the window of an antique store in Sydney, Australia, and it made me think that perhaps that old hand-me-down instrument, too, could be seen as an antique. My cousin had long ago consigned it to the attic of his house and was happy to return it to me. Patient application of polish revealed that, sure enough, the microscope wasn't black—it was brass and could be made to shine. It was an antique! It was only later that I learned to forgo the polishing of old instruments.

On my travels over the ensuing decades, I kept an eye out for antique, or at least fairly old, microscopes. I did not hunt them on the internet, or try to track them down through specialty dealers. I liked buying them at flea-markets, junk stores and all-purpose country antique shops. The fun was in the chance encounter. Eventually there were 35 microscopes in my collection, and I enjoyed making a detailed examination of each one, making a record of its design, optics, accessories and provenance, and I derive great pleasure from seeing them displayed among the books on our library shelves at home.

An unexpected off-shoot of collecting old microscopes was a rewarding correspondence with a school-teacher in England, Donald C. Bruce. Through some historical organisation, he and I were on record as being interested in microscopes and old books about microscopy. We exchanged letters through the 1970s and '80s. Occasionally we helped each other out by sending a wanted book. We were not dealing with valuable antiquities and worked on the tacit assumption that our modest expenditures would roughly balance out over time.

For me, the most interesting feature of this exchange turned out to be Bruce's experience in World War II. As Sergeant Don Bruce, he had been navigator on the crew of a Lancaster bomber of the Royal Air Force. When his aircraft was shot down over Belgium, the crew bailed out safely, and Bruce spent the rest of the war in Germany, as a prisoner-of-war. Interspersed among his letters to me about scientific instruments were fascinating accounts of time spent in the prison camp. Some of these accounts were sent to me as tape-recordings housed in cassettes.

Eventually, Don Bruce's interest became focused more on antique mechanical devices, especially calculating machines, and our correspondence fizzled out. Now near the end of life I find myself confronted not only with disposing of a great many books and papers and assorted things, but also with the challenge of disposing of a microscope collection. Disposal of the Bruce correspondence and tape cassettes was easier—I gave them to the RAF Museum in London.

A love of teaching

My teaching had begun while I was at the Merck labs. Much of it was in the form of university seminars, but as an adjunct professor at the University of Pennsylvania I gave periodic lectures at its school of veterinary medicine.

More significant, because more regular, and covering a much longer period of time, was my appointment as an adjunct professor at New York College of Medicine. For 25 consecutive years, I gave a series of autumn lectures on human helminthology—a course popularly known as 'the worm lectures'. The series came about because Soldano Ferrone, chair of microbiology and immunology at NYCM consulted Merck Research management about finding someone who could teach parasitology to medical students.

On their recommendation he hired me, sight unseen. When I showed up for the first series of lectures, he shared his time, his thoughts, and his office-space, and did everything humanly possible to make me feel welcome. Over the following quarter century, I was similarly welcomed—generously and warmly—by members of the department, especially Doctors Ferrone, Wasserman, Bucher, Geliebter, Mordue and Schwartz.

The typically modest academic fee that I was paid for these lectures was certainly not the motivation for the effort I put into this work—and it was a lot of work, because the preparation of up-to-date illustrated lectures was not part of my 'day job'. My motivation was the happiness I derived from interaction with, and evident appreciation by, the students and faculty of the college. As I said much later, on the occasion of receiving the NYMC William Cullen Bryant Award: 'In the early days, my lectures were in early winter and I often drove up from New Jersey in very wintry weather. As I drove, I would ask myself "why am I doing this?" On the way back, I knew the answer!'

At Drew University, I began to teach undergraduate courses on the biology of parasitic diseases, and in the Caspersen School of Graduate Studies I taught the history of biomedical science.

I enjoyed teaching medical history to mature and highly motivated students, not only for the sheer fun of doing it, but also because it was a strong motivator for me to continue to develop my expertise in the subject. The course was 'History of biomedical science', because I did not wish to deal with the social and political aspects of the history of the medical profession. Another great stimulus was my participation in the History of Medicine Society of New Jersey. I enjoyed its meetings even though it involved travel to Princeton, where the meetings were held. My amateur status in the field added zest to my participation as a member (and later president) of the society and to my being presented the society's David L. Cowan Award for Achievements in Medical History.

I often recall a conversation I had at a cocktail party in our neighbourhood in New Jersey around the time I started at Drew. I happened to start chatting to a professor of English from Rutgers University, and our conversation soon became animated on both sides. We were both excited: he because he was retiring from teaching and I because I was starting teaching. It was a neat, complementary exchange.

For me, getting to teach was one of the big joys in my life. I had been influenced by so many of my own teachers and mentors—my tutor Miss Martin, my biology teacher Robert Wells at Campbell College and then J.D. Smyth at Trinity College Dublin, who instilled in me such a love of parasite biology—and now it was to be my turn.

When I started, I felt very much at home in my parasitology courses, but I felt that I was almost an imposter in the context of teaching the history of medicine, but I kept going for twenty years because I loved it. I supervised a few graduate theses on the history of medicine. One doctoral student, Sherrilyn Sethi, has recorded how my lecture on Andreas Vesalius influenced her choice of career by leading her to specialise in medical humanities—and to positions of responsibility at the University of Massachusetts Medical School.

I can understand how professors burn out after years of teaching, but for me it was the perfect combination: I was teaching material that I wanted to teach, and because it was quite specialised, the students were generally there because they wanted to be. I didn't have to do other teaching to justify my position, so the situation was pretty much ideal.

Beyond the classroom, mentoring had its own component of teaching. Many of the students that I mentored returned for my Drew retirement 'do' in 2010, and even spoke at the event. I was touched by that, and very glad to see them. It was also gratifying to hear from absent students who had appreciated my work with them—I remember a very moving note from the mother of one of the students saying how my mentorship had changed her daughter's life.

At that stage, Mary and I moved from our house in New Jersey to a retirement community in Massachusetts. That move away from New Jersey, where we had spent so many happy years, was not easy. I gave away a lot of books. I threw away a lot of printed papers (they are mostly online now, no need to store them on paper). Our new community is vibrant and full of activity. We devoted our time to getting to know people and exchanging visits with family members. I continued to keep an eye out for professional opportunities, and got involved in local committee work. Opportunities for walking, hiking, snow-shoeing, kayaking and that sort of thing seemed limitless.

Then, in October 2015, any notion of a quiet retirement quickly vanished.

Stockholm, Sweden

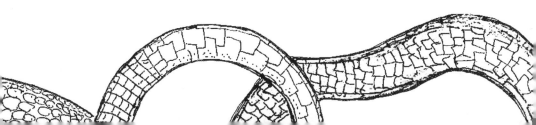

Chaos and Bagpipes—the Nobel Prize

I have often been asked if I was surprised about getting the Nobel prize. There are a couple of answers to that. Yes, I was personally very surprised. In some ways the situation felt awkward, because the enormous impact of ivermectin in human and veterinary medicine had resulted from an extraordinary effort involving many people. There had been scattered public suggestions that the discovery of ivermectin was prizeworthy; traditionally though, the Nobel prize (apart from the Peace Prize) is not awarded to groups of more than three persons, and it would be hard to select only three in this case. Still, if three were to be chosen, it was certainly possible that I would be one of them. I had been elected to the US National Academy of Sciences. I had many publications to my credit and was well-known in my field of science. I had initiated the investigation of the potential role of ivermectin for the control of heartworm disease in dogs and the much more 'high-profile' investigation of the potential role of ivermectin in the control of river blindness. (On the other hand, I had just published an account of the ivermectin discovery that would illustrate 'the limited role played by an individual in this supremely team-oriented endeavor'.)

Earlier, a Merck executive who had just joined the company commented that the discovery of ivermectin might someday be worthy of a Nobel prize. At the time we thought that was a hoot, we weren't thinking that way. On the other hand, a distinguished professor of veterinary medicine had told me at a conference that he had nominated me for the Nobel prize and was gathering support for a campaign to make it happen. I dismissed the idea out of hand. Indeed, I was so dismissive and derisive about it, that I telephoned him about a week later to apologise for being so brusque and for not even thanking him for his generous impulse on my behalf.

These factors were in the background, yet I was oblivious to the impending announcement. I did not then know that there was a consistent season of the year for Nobel announcements—never mind a particular day in December for the actual award ceremony.

Then I got the call. Not the call from a representative of the Nobel Committee in Stockholm, but a slightly earlier call from a journalist. It was early on a morning in October. I got to the phone and the journalist told me I had won the Nobel prize. At that exact moment, it was a surprise—a very big surprise. I actually said to him 'You have to be kidding' and he replied that it was true and that I could check the Nobel.org website. I did, right away, and sure enough, there it was. The Nobel Committee had chosen to recognise the importance of ivermectin with a Nobel prize and they had chosen me as a recipient. That announcement, I knew right away, was going to change things!

The official call from Stockholm came a little later and reassured me that the whole thing was not a dream. Apparently, communication across time-zones leads to difficulties in getting the word to new Nobel recipients. My co-recipients, Professor Tu in China and Professor Ōmura in Japan, may have been more awake when they heard the news.

But back in Massachusetts at our house that morning, Mary and I soon found ourselves in the middle of a happy, chaotic storm. We had reporters gathering outside and then inside the house. Neighbours were emerging from front doors to see what was going on. Everyone was excited. Then suddenly we heard the skirl of bagpipes. Maybe this was a dream after all? Reporters who had a minute ago been bombarding me with questions were now streaming outside to find the source of such stirring sound. I followed them. Almost immediately I encountered a famous cancer paediatrician from a famous Boston hospital. Was he coming to congratulate me as a neighbour from up the street? Or was he, you might ask, one of the crowd trying to locate the bagpiper? No, he was the bagpiper. Friends though we were, I don't think I spoke a word to him on that occasion (who would dare to interfere with a piper piping?). Cheerful chaos all around!

We started getting messages from everyone, including a Merck chemist, a leader on the ivermectin project. He was originally from Germany and had gone camping in the Black Forest, only to emerge into civilisation and be greeted by the news of his old colleague, the worm guy, getting the Nobel prize!

The volume of calls flooding in meant that our own children couldn't get through to us. Jenifer had been trying to call and, when she got to the school where she taught, she eventually got through to me and I confirmed the news. The school assembly was in full swing and the headmaster asked her to come up and tell everyone what had just happened, then she started to get calls from media seeking interviews. By this time, Betsy had seen the news on CNN, and had sent me an email with multiple exclamation marks. The family excitement was deeply meaningful and helped me cope with the news.

Throughout the day, the magnitude of the whole thing was hitting me. But there was also an element of regret and unease regarding my colleagues. Would my name be mud now? There were reasons why I was selected for the Nobel prize, but there would have been reasons for selecting other people too. That didn't soften the reality of the fact that so many excellent people had been part of this discovery, but could not share the prize.

My fears were eased over time as individual colleagues congratulated me with messages of genuine warmth. Then, a short time after the announcement, Merck organised an event to celebrate the prize. Many of the people who had worked closely with me at Merck sat right up at the front of the packed lecture theatre, and as I walked in I received an enormously enthusiastic expression of support. For me, this was one of the most emotional moments of the entire Nobel prize experience, and when I recall it, I still feel that flood of warm collegiality and friendship. Had I the chance to re-live one day from that period, that might be it.

Dealing with excessive credit

Some years ago, scholarly attention was directed towards 'The Matthew effect'—the application to everyday-life of the biblical maxim (Book of Matthew) that 'For whoever has, to him more shall be given…'. The label was coined by Robert Merton, with particular reference to the observation that scientists with many honours tend to accumulate further honours at a higher rate than do scientists with few honours. It does sometimes seem that people who receive awards are given additional awards at a disproportionately high rate. In many cases the apparent effect is undoubtedly an illusion, but I sometimes feel that I might be an innocent victim, or an undeserving beneficiary, of something akin to the Matthew Effect.

As speaker, I am from time to time introduced as the discoverer of ivermectin. I am then obliged to point out, early in my talk, that neither I nor anyone else can justly be called the discoverer of ivermectin. People sometimes attribute my rejection of the 'discoverer' title to modesty. But it is not a matter of modesty. It is a matter of duty, decorum and discomfort. Of these, the primary motivator is probably discomfort. It is the one that is least optional. It is impossible for me to overlook the team aspect of the discovery. I do not have to launch into a discussion of the team on every occasion, but I do have to acknowledge that the discovery was the result of teamwork.

I suspect that there must be a universal desire to bestow awards—gifts, too, perhaps but that's a different matter; you cannot earn a gift. A particular award might be tantamount to a gift, but the more it becomes a gift the less it becomes an award. What awards and gifts have in common is the plain fact that, unless a genuine ethical principle is at stake, their refusal makes the refuser feel churlish and makes the giver feel slighted. These musings are undoubtedly an attempt on my part to further excuse my neglect of a cultural inheritance that urges me to deflect or disparage a compliment of any kind.

Something I have learned through experience in recent years is that a rejection or down-playing of credit is a 'downer' for the audience. This applies to personal conversation as well as to public speech. One way to diminish this dampening effect is to hold back from jumping in and correcting or modulating a remark that gives one too much credit for some particular aspect of discovery. Inevitably one comes to respond by swallowing hard and letting it pass.

Have others experienced this reluctance to constantly correct? I suspect that this was the source of much criticism of Sir Alexander Fleming regarding the discovery of penicillin. He never claimed credit to which he was not entitled, but he was accused of failing to contradict remarks that gave him too much credit. Thus, he gained a reputation for unseemly basking in public adulation. That reputation may be well founded. On the other hand, it may be completely false. Until recently I would not have presumed to take a position on the matter. Accounts of his life suggest a personality inconsistent with excessive glory-seeking. He may simply have found it easier to 'go with the flow' than to disappoint his admirers by disparaging their accolades. I draw no comparison between Fleming's career and mine, but on the basis of my own experience of dealing with excess credit, I am inclined to give Fleming the benefit of the doubt on this matter.

The road to Stockholm

When someone asks me where I am from, my answer is slightly complicated. I was born in Londonderry, in the United Kingdom, but within days, was brought back across the border to my family home in County Donegal, Ireland. That is where I spent my childhood, except for periods at boarding school in Portrush and Belfast. I have held Irish and Northern Irish driving licences, and Irish and British passports; but I have lived and worked for most of my life in the United States of America, and I am a US citizen.

The riddle of where I am from has neither impinged upon nor troubled me for much of my life, but it did present a conundrum when I was announced as a recipient of the Nobel prize. The question came up—which country's embassy in Sweden would look after me for the Nobel prize ceremony? Ultimately, it was the USA's embassy that took me under its wing. But before we got anywhere near Stockholm, the Swedish and Norwegian embassies in the USA helped Mary and me prepare.

All four American laureates of 2015 were put through our paces at a dinner hosted by both ambassadors and held at the residence of the Swedish ambassador in Washington, D.C. At that dinner, Norwegian and Swedish comperes asked each of us questions as individuals and we had to answer the question in very little time. I remember getting to my feet trying to think of something to say. If it didn't come to me right away I was dead in the water! Very publicly! It was a challenging interlude but it was all done with humour and in a friendly atmosphere. Going through these exercises was extremely helpful, as it prepared us for the ceremonies to come. At the same dinner, I sat beside a Rear Admiral in the US Navy who was in full-dress uniform. She was in the US public health service (the military connection going back to the quarantining of ships when cholera and other dread fevers were rampant). She was concerned about the need for more publicity for the great, much neglected, tropical diseases. This was an interesting perspective for me, because in my field I am constantly aware of the great tropical diseases; they are part of my life. During dessert, her husband, a US senator, stopped by for a chat. Because of the Scandinavian background of the dinner-party, spouses were not seated at the same table as their partners, and this, too, was excellent preparation for social events to come.

On another occasion, Mary and I were invited to the White House to meet President Barack Obama. This was a big deal, and it, too, was organised by the Norwegian and Swedish embassies in Washington, D.C. Again, the invitation was extended to all four American laureates and their spouses. There was, of course, tremendous security around the White House, and various paths to be navigated and checkpoints to be passed. Mary needed a little help getting around, and she had a wheelchair for that. One of the scenes I love to recall from that day is my memory of the Swedish ambassador pushing Mary along in the wheelchair. He and his wife were wonderful hosts, as were all the Swedish and Norwegian embassy representatives. Being inside the White House is not the same as being in the West Wing. Being in the West Wing is not the same as being in the Oval Office. On the way to that inner sanctum of American presidents, the four American Nobel laureates and their wives were shepherded from room to room getting closer and closer to our destination.

We chatted casually to each other and to our White House escorts, sometimes pausing to look at interesting historical paintings on the wall. It was 10 November 2015, and in anterooms and corridors, aides and functionaries hurried about with an air of serious intent. From time to time we were given updates as to when exactly we might be face to face with the president. There was a sense of eager anticipation in the air, but some anxiety, too. Everyone was acutely aware that the presidential schedule is subject to delay, or even cancellation at any moment. It was like waiting at the doctor's office—but not exactly the same!

The four American laureates were Paul Modrich (born in the USA), Angus Deaton (born in Scotland), Aziz Sancar (born in Turkey), and me (born in Northern Ireland). We and our spouses had just met that morning and were enjoying getting to know each other. And of course we were showing absolutely no outward trace of excitement! On finally entering the Oval Office each couple, in turn, was introduced to the president. When he was talking to Mary and me, he suddenly put his hand in his pocket and pulled out a present for me. This was most unusual, none of the others were getting a present. But he handed me a little stuffed animal representing a dog heartworm! That was really special. I still have it, this little plush toy with an embroidered heart on it.

When all four laureate couples had been introduced to the president, we mingled in the area in front of his desk and enjoyed a bit of informal chatting with each other and with the Norwegian and Swedish ambassadors and their wives. At one point the laureates stood in a line and President Obama gave us a little congratulatory talk. Indeed, in congratulating us on our Nobel prizes he added parenthetically that he was still trying to earn the one he had himself received (having been awarded the Peace Prize in 2009). Aziz Sancar surprised us all by asking if he might ask a question, and got an immediate 'yes.' The question was about how more funds could be made available for biomedical research and Obama rose to the occasion without batting an eye. Clearly, he was well informed and perfectly able to address the topic.

But for me there was a question that remained unanswered. The president could not be expected to be familiar with the details of the work done by each Nobel laureate. How, then, had it come about that the president of the United States should suddenly pull a dog heartworm from his pocket? OK, it was just a fuzzy model of a heartworm—but still, he must have been told that the strange gift would symbolise a central focus of my research on the drug ivermectin. Who had told him that?

As Mary and I had entered the Oval Office, we had been introduced to the president by one of the scientists and science-policy experts from the Office of the President's Science Advisor. Although we had been introduced to that young woman (and had a delightful chat in her office upon leaving the Oval Office) I must confess that I left the White House without realising that she might have been responsible for the heartworm gift. In one of those once-in a-million coincidences, one of my children is married to someone who is acquainted with someone who (we later discovered) is a sister of that young woman. So, I now know that, for that memorable gift of the fluffy white 'worm', I am indebted both to President Barack Obama and to Dr Jo Handelsman, an eminent parasitologist, now director of the Wisconsin Institute for Discovery at the University of Wisconsin-Madison.

That meeting with President Obama was special in itself, but having a picture of Mary and me meeting him in the White House has gone on to have another kind of impact—one that I have seen when talking to young students. As an example, in the community where I live, we have many medical experts, and sometimes inner-city school students come in to learn about healthcare occupations and hear from people who have worked as surgeons, general practitioners, nurses' aides, therapists and so forth. I talk to them about my work as a researcher and how it led to the Nobel prize. When I show a photo of the meeting with the King and the Queen of Sweden they may be impressed; but when I show a photo of the meeting with President Obama, they gasp. The king and queen are not part of their lives. President Obama is.

The Stockholm experience

There is something special about the phrase 'going to the palace'. Even the most fervent egalitarian mind, the most ardent anti-monarchist heart, is likely to feel a nudge upon receiving an invitation from 'Their Majesties the King and Queen'—an invitation to have dinner at their place. That is the sort of thing that makes the Nobel celebration in Stockholm a kind of fairy-tale. Still, it is a mere highlight and is only a small part of the week-long experience.

It begins at the airport. Well, actually it begins well before that. Between the announcement in October and arrival in Stockholm in early December there are preparations to be made. If you are a Nobel laureate, you will, most fortunately, be put in touch right away with one particular person at the Nobel Foundation in Sweden who will guide you through the maze of preparations and planning. This will include the sorting-out of various extra-Nobel functions, such as invitations to speak at universities (and decisions about which you will accept); and decisions about guests (of which a maximum number is specified for any given year). Forms must be filled out and sent to Stockholm. Promises must be made—that you will give a Nobel lecture, for example. Preferences must be recorded and details submitted, as to travel, rental of formal attire for you and your guests; security matters (nationality of each guest).

Then there is Stockholm in December! The Nobel prizes are always given in December, because Alfred Nobel died on the tenth of that month in 1896. Some of his modern compatriots mildly suggest that it was inconsiderate of him to depart this world at that particular time—of wintry conditions, difficult travel and little daylight. But that is how it is, and the attention of the Nobel organisation (and much of Sweden!) is annually focussed on 10 December. On the brighter side, Stockholm is ablaze with tiny white lights during those many hours of darkness. The trees, buildings, statues and other objects are festooned with white lights, creating the perfect setting for the 'fairytale' that is the Nobel experience.

At the airport in Stockholm, Mary and I were greeted by Urban Lendahl of the Karolinska Institute, who served as secretary-general of the institute's Nobel Committee for the prize in physiology or medicine, as well as being secretary-general of the Nobel Assembly (50 Karolinska-based professors who determine the eventual winners in that category).

He immediately made us feel welcome, and he continued to do so as we spent time with him throughout our stay in Stockholm. He introduced us to two others with whom we would spend even more time—Jan Mattson who would be our driver for the next eight-days, and Filippa Briggs, our attaché for that period. They were wonderful people, and, given the extensive and variable demands of the Nobel schedule, their spouses were undoubtedly wonderful, too. Filippa was one of a cadre of attachés who spoke whatever language needed to be spoken, and solved whatever problem needed to be solved. Filippa was the only person in the whole world who knew just where Mary and I should be at any time, and what we should be doing (or not doing)—as well as knowing just how to make sure, tactfully and gracefully, that we would in fact be in the proper place and doing what we were supposed to be doing. It seems to be a standing joke in Nobel circles that when laureates finally depart for home, they have a longing to take their attachés and drivers with them. We can identify with that sentiment!

During Nobel Week, Stockholm's Grand Hotel sets aside a special space for the Nobel Desk. One cannot help suspecting that without the Nobel Desk the world would come to an end before the week has ended. Its charming attendants seem to have but one response to any problem brought to them: 'Leave it to us'.

Mary had beautiful, silvery shoes to go with her beautiful blue evening gown. The shoes had very smooth, slick soles, and we had heard that the floors of the Royal Palace are polished to a very slippery finish. This was a bit of a worry, and on the morning of the Royal Banquet we took the shoes to the Nobel Desk and told them of our concern. They said 'Leave it to us'.

When we returned some hours later, the shoes had been returned by a Stockholm cobbler, perfectly equipped with thin leather soles—and Mary was able to tread the Royal Floor with confidence (and they all lived happily ever after and …).

Because of the White House visit, as well as the US embassy reception and other activities in Stockholm, Mary and I had had very-welcome opportunities to spend some time with the other American laureates and their wives, and to get to know them a little. Getting to know the 2015 laureates from other countries was more challenging, partly because of language barriers and partly because all us were busy interacting with our own families, friends, colleagues and compatriots. I would have been interested in talking to Belorusian author Svetlana Alexievich, Nobel laureate in Literature, but she and I did not share a language. Her writings on Chernobyl and other tragedies can seem inexpressibly grim, but in a panel discussion she pointed out (through interpreters) that her subject in those writings was not disaster, but love. It was an insight that transforms the experience of reading her works.

At one point a press-conference was held for the three 'medicine' laureates, Professor Ōmura from Japan, Professor Tu from China, and myself. Professor Ōmura was known to the Japanese reporters in Stockholm, and some of them were eager to talk to me informally because Professor Ōmura and I were co-recipients of a share of the 2015 medicine prize (Professor Tu had been awarded a separate share). They were surprised to learn that Professor Ōmura and I had met on only one previous occasion. It was in 1999 when I was giving a series of lectures at Japanese institutions, including the Kitasato Institute in Tokyo, where Professor Ōmura was my host.

Pomp and Ceremony—A Nobel week

Before I had any reason to think too much about the Nobel prize, I suppose I assumed the ceremony in Stockholm took about a half day and that was it. That's the part you see on the television, when the prizes are given to the recipients. As soon as I heard I had won though, I realised there was a lot more to it than that! The organisational activities began almost immediately, and there were lots of instructions about dress codes and invitations and the choreography for the various banquets and concerts and activities that would take place over the course of a week in Stockholm.

During our time there, Mary required a little assistance in getting around, as I was needed to be in particular places at particular venues and not always able to be by her side. For the Royal Procession down the grand staircase at the beginning of the Nobel Banquet, she had a tall, young Swedish man to accompany her and lend an arm to ensure her safety on the stairs. Also, because Mary needed to use elevators rather than stairs, it meant we got to see a lot of parts of places that others did not, as the elevators were often away from the public parts of the building. It was sometimes a challenge to cope with the autograph hunters, who would cluster at the entrance of a building and were apt to be unduly importunate. So Mary would enter a building with our driver, Jan, and I would enter with Filippa, our attaché. Our Swedish 'partners' would deftly and diplomatically get us through.

Getting to the Nobel award ceremony was almost as exciting as being there. Jan wore his official cap and badge to drive us to the event, and we were in our finery. Our limousine was well positioned in a line of identical black limousines parked in front of the Grand Hotel. Of these, ten were for the laureate couples, and five were for special dignitaries. At the appointed time, we set off in an orderly line, with an escort of many identical police motorcycles with flashing lights. Some, perhaps all, of the riders were women. We proceeded slowly through the centre of Stockholm, while the darkening December afternoon was wildly punctuated by white Christmas lights and the flashing yellow lights of the motorcycles. I noticed the side streets conspicuously closed off and filled with traffic, waiting for the retinue to pass by. For me, that short journey in an escorted motorcade was one of the most thrilling aspects of the whole week.

The prize-giving ceremony itself was magical. My wife, our daughters with their husbands, and my brother Bert with his wife Anne, were in the audience. As laureates, we had been instructed as to the direction in which we should face, and when to bow, and how to receive the prize from the king of Sweden onstage. When it was my turn, I was focused on the choreography, stepping forward and back and bowing and turning in the correct order. So focused was I, that I have no idea what I said to the king in those moments, nor what he said to me. But I am told by my family that the whole thing went smoothly, and they cheered accordingly.

Once the formal part was over, people thronged the stage, family and friends mingled, it was a great hullabaloo! The provost of Trinity College Dublin, Patrick Prendergast, was there, which was a lovely surprise, and, at my invitation, the former CEO of Merck, Roy Vagelos, and his wife were also present. It was a truly special gathering. At one point, I realised that I no longer had the medal with me. There was no need to panic. The level of organisation was such that the Nobel staff, in their expert way, had unobtrusively taken the medals from the laureates without even disturbing their conversations, and the medals were to be kept safe and returned to us at the end of the week.

And what a week it was. One of the many highlights was a visit to the Royal Palace and getting to meet its primary occupants. A specific time was set aside just for that. A portion of the 'Princes Gallery' had been screened off, and each couple (Nobel laureate and spouse) was, in turn, escorted into that space and introduced to their majesties, King Carl XVI Gustaf and Queen Silvia. The escorts quietly withdrew to some distance, leaving a happy foursome to have a chat. After the initial exchange of handshakes and pleasantries, I found myself talking to the king while Mary talked with the queen.

At one point, I brought up the subject of Carolus Linnaeus, the great eighteenth-century Swedish biologist, whose name is immortalised by the letter 'L' in numerous Latin biological names. He had long been prominent in my interest in the history of biology; before leaving home, I had skimmed through my old copy of Goerke's biography. His Majesty adroitly steered the conversation to the more pertinent topic of today's young Swedish scientists. Mary and Queen Silvia had a relaxed chat.

Also notable was a banquet hosted by the Nobel Committee of the Karolinska Institute in honour of the 2015 laureates in physiology or medicine. It was held in a former prince's palace, elegant in architecture and décor, with culinary art to match— even the menus were enfolded within works of art. It gave us a welcome chance to converse with those most directly responsible for our awards. It was particularly interesting to talk to Juleen R. Zierath, chair of the Karolinska Institute's Nobel Committee, and the already mentioned Urban Lendahl. Earlier, Dr Lendahl had taken us to visit the room where, every October, the 50 members of the Nobel Assembly sit around a table (a very large round table!) to finalise their decision and immediately announce it to the public. We were told that we had been under scrutiny for several years, presumably to assure us that we had not been the beneficiaries of a momentary whim.

That was by no means the end of banqueting. After the award ceremony on 10 December, Mary and I and our guests attended the Nobel Banquet, a feast for 1,300 seated guests, where we sat at the table of honour and were entertained by musical interludes, artistic lighting displays and short speeches. For one of the speeches it fell to my lot to express thanks on behalf of the laureates in physiology or medicine. Brevity was critical, and provided a welcome challenge in drafting the speech. (That brevity also makes it feasible to reproduce the text of my speech in this volume.) I was careful to refrain from thanking King Carl Gustaf, for he was a fellow guest, so to speak, on that occasion.

His Majesty was, however, host rather than guest on the following evening at a magnificent banquet at the Royal Palace. Some 800 guests sat at one astonishingly long table, and each couple had a dedicated footman. Mary sat beside the prime minister of Sweden while I was beside Princess Sophia. We both had wonderfully animated and enjoyable conversations with our dinner companions—as we had had with other guests during the preliminary reception period.

On another evening there was a wonderful concert, featuring the young Russian pianist Daniil Trifonov. He played Rachmaninoff's famously virtuosic Third piano concerto. It was not only good to hear, but for people like me who are musically challenged, it was good to watch—a brilliant and flamboyant performer with hands flying and forelock jumping as he bounced up and down! It was amazing. A high-powered concerto to grace a high-powered week.

Speech from the Nobel Banquet, Stockholm, 10 December 2015

Your Majesties, Your Royal Highnesses, Your Excellencies, Ladies and Gentlemen,

I speak on behalf of Professor Tu, Professor Ōmura and myself, in saying that we wish to thank Karolinska Institute and the members of its committee who found our work worthy of such generous, and conspicuous, recognition. And we thank the members of the Nobel Foundation—especially those who made possible today's splendid award ceremony and banquet.

Professor Tu, Professor Ōmura and I come from different lands. We speak with different tongues. But we are as one in gratitude.

Actually, we have something else in common. All three of us have been connected, one way or another, with the world of parasites. Professor Tu and Professor Ōmura work on microorganisms that are very important—but they are very small. I like something bigger. Worm parasites are a decent size. Worms are something you can really get your teeth into.

Parasites are not generally regarded as being loveable. When we refer to some people as parasites, we are not being complimentary; we are not praising them. We think that a parasite is the sort of person who goes through a revolving-door on somebody else's push. It is so unfair! Unfair to the real parasites—the innumerable and influential parasites of the natural world. Your Majesties, Your Royal Highnesses, Your Excellencies, Ladies and Gentlemen it is time for parasites to get a little more respect!

And it is with much respect that we end, as we began, with our thanks to you. We add that we are grateful also to those who made our work possible, those who made our lives possible, and those who make our lives worth living. To all of you and all of them we say, Thank you.

'What did you do with the money?'

Almost nobody has asked me how much money I got for the Nobel prize, or what I did with it. People feel it is impolite to pry. No such social constraints held back a primary-school student in County Meath, Ireland, from asking me. This girl, aged about six, asked with admirable candour 'How much money did you get with the prize'. The adults in the room were suitably shocked and amused, but I was happy to reply.

Bearing in mind that the prize was divided among three recipients, that I spent a bit of my share for expenses in Stockholm, and that the US Internal Revenue Service took a large chunk of it in taxes, my take-home was about $230,000.

Since I was not able to share the Nobel medal or the prize money with colleagues at Merck, I shared the money among organisations devoted to the assistance of students, especially in the field of biomedical science. Others, too, made generous donations in honour of the prize—some were given to Drew University by parents of my former students.

When I returned to Ireland in 2016 and 2017, many kind people held celebrations. There was an unforgettable 'big bash' in my home-town of Ramelton. Various institutions around the country hosted events, including the Royal Irish Academy; Trinity College Dublin; Queen's University, Belfast; the Institute of Technology, Sligo; Campbell College, Belfast; Letterkenny University Hospital; and the University of Ulster; as well as many primary and secondary schools. With other honourees, I received the President's Award from the hands of President of Ireland Michael D. Higgins.

Mind your language

Since sharing the Nobel prize I have done many interviews, and I am generally careful about how I phrase things. On occasion though, I have been unwise with words.

During an interview in 2016 with Patricia Harty, the distinguished editor of *Irish America Magazine*, I said that the chairman and CEO of Merck had decided 'in collusion' with a handful of top associates to donate ivermectin for the treatment of river blindness in humans. That was back when I thought that 'collusion' simply meant putting heads together.

When I read the interview in print, something didn't feel quite right about my wording. I found that 'collusion' always has a negative connotation. One doesn't collude for good! I should, of course, have written 'in collaboration'. In conversation, such mistakes can be quickly amended and hopefully laughed off without offence. But in print, I felt it needed a clarification, and the October/November 2016 edition of *Irish America Magazine* carried it thus:

> There is, I think something especially appealing in the idea of corporate executives huddling together and plotting to implement a good deed of that magnitude. The Merck CEO, Dr Roy Vagelos, has himself said that he neglected even to inform the Merck board of directors that he was about to commit the company to that extraordinary action.
>
> Nevertheless, readers may see something sinister in my flippant use of the word 'collusion'. I would like to assure readers of my unalloyed admiration, then and now, for the decision and the decision makers. My disclaimer of a personal role in the decision was not intended to distance myself from something bad, but rather to acknowledge that I was not a member of the small group of executives who decided in favor of something good!

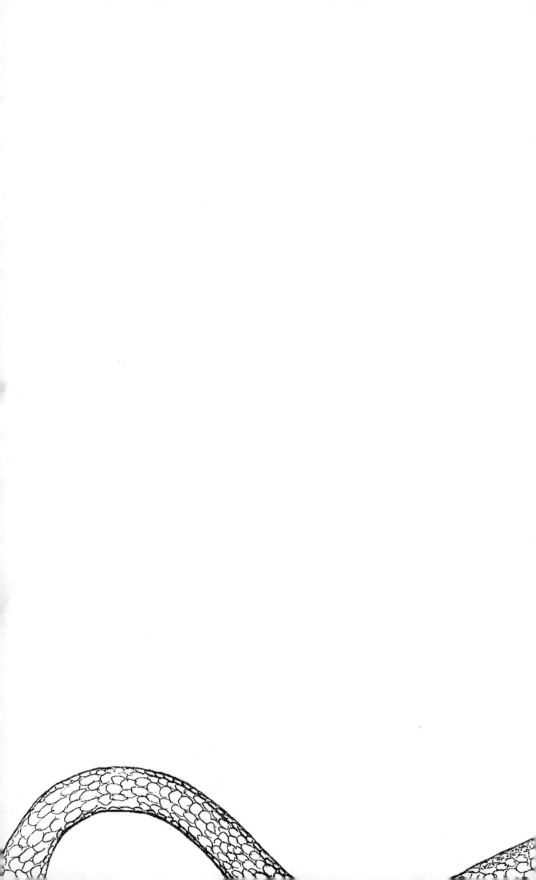

Things learned
along the way

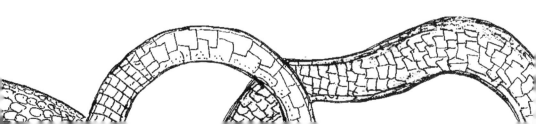

Be prepared

A consequence of becoming a Nobel laureate is that one becomes subject to interrogation on matters quite unlimited in their irrelevance to one's experience. Still, coming to the end of this long screed, and nearing what must be the end of this long life, it is perhaps fitting to set down a few parting remarks about things I might have learned, or should have learned. I have no special qualification for such an exercise. What I do have is an invitation to try it in this space—and that is an invitation I am incapable of refusing.

While a life of excessive preparation is to be deplored, preparation in itself is, of course, to be applauded—especially in areas in which it seems to be in short supply. In the world of public speaking, there are those who seem to regard the very idea of preparation as an affront to the efficient use of their precious time. In exchanges with friends, they may be morally free (but not necessarily wise) to say what they please. But when it comes to public communication, they should have a little care for the rest of us and our precious time. Nobody doubts their ability to 'wing it'. (Okay, I often doubt it, but that is not the point.) Preparation will encourage you to be cautious about using satire (it is good only in the hands of a master orator); to be scrupulous in avoiding sarcasm (always bad in public communication); and to devise a strong ending. The point is that in public speaking, preparation is a good investment.

A more specific thing that bugs me about ill-prepared speech is the common lackadaisical manner of introducing a speaker. An introduction does not have to be stern. It can be joyful, but it must be free of shilly-shallying. Surely it is not too much to ask that an introduction from the podium should follow a few basic principles: (1) Include the title or subject-matter of the talk; keep silent about what the speaker is going to say. (2) Include the speaker's name and essential qualification for being the speaker; keep silent as to whether the speaker is known to be eloquent or funny or to possess other virtues as a speaker. (3) Include an ending in the form of a welcoming call on the speaker to speak; then keep silent. Departure from any one of these precepts is likely to place both the speaker and the audience at a disadvantage. Such departure will constitute a discourtesy, however unintentional, toward speaker and listener.

Lucky escapes

In the course of a long life, one comes to realise that there is a very fine line between good luck and bad luck. Most of us, late in life, will probably be able to recall encounters that could have had disastrous consequences—but did not.

My childhood in Ramelton offered some memorable moments of peril. In a storehouse loft behind the house, we had a home-made swing tied to the rafters with barn rope. I remember frequently going up to play on that swing by myself. It was a long rope, and you could get a long pendulum going on it. But one day, it broke when I was using it. Looking back at my life I see that I had some narrow escapes, and this was one. The rope broke when the swing was past the midpoint but not at the top. I came straight down and landed in a yoga-sitting position, completely unhurt. If I had come down on my head, I might not be here.

One of our favourite destinations for family outings was a secluded, and then often deserted, beach called the Kinnegar, which lay beyond Rathmullan. I remember my father once saying that he had lain awake at night because he was thinking of the previous day when he had been swimming with us at the Kinnegar. The tide had come in over sandbars, placing my siblings and me out of our depth, and he had instructed us to swim immediately toward the beach. I think this must have been memorable because, seen in hindsight, it would have been my earliest insight into parenthood. For me, as a child, it had just been a little bit of excitement; now I was struck by the more grown-up realisation that for my father it had been different.

As an aside, another lucky escape springs to mind from a little later in life. In my college days in Dublin, it was fairly common for people in a hurry to run after a city bus as it was leaving a bus stop, and to jump onto its open rear platform while grabbing the vertical metal pole placed there to aid passengers alighting or boarding the bus. I tried it once. The bus was moving away from the bus stop rapidly, and I, lacking experience, did not provide the proper amount of forward momentum to ensure a safe footing on the rear platform. I did not fall. My forward foot landed on the edge of the platform, but far enough forward on the surface to carry my weight, with just my heel overhanging the edge. No damage at all. But, oh the damage that might have ensued had my foot been a couple of inches to the rear. My grip of the pole would have stretched my forward-moving body toward the horizontal position, and the resultant injuries could have maimed me for life, or ended my life. A lesson on how not to board a bus was learned in an instant. That was useful, yet seemed somehow trivial even then. But the enormity of the difference between what-was and what-might-have-been was a realisation so unsettling that the bus incident still haunts my adult 'memory-box'.

These episodes are more or less simple physical affairs. Others have a social rather than a physical basis. They are more hauntingly significant because they could so easily have belonged to a broader category that might be termed 'Lives Wrongly Ruined'. One such close call came about through shopping. It was the early 1970s, and I was in a hardware store in Liverpool, New South Wales, buying nails and screws and other small items such as might be needed for minor household repairs. Some were destined for our Australian home, which was the director's residence at the Merck Sharp & Dohme Veterinary Research Laboratory. Other items would be used for 'fix-it' jobs on our furniture, toys and other personal property that would eventually be taken back to the USA. I kept the two groups separate, in order to exclude the personal items from the routine list of reimbursable work-related expenses. There must have been only two or three items in each category, because I held them in front of me, one category each hand. Then, lost in thought, I walked blithely and innocently out of the shop. I was several yards away when a man approached from behind and, quietly catching up with me, said 'Did you want to pay for those items, Sir?' We walked back to the shop, where the situation was easily cleared up.

But imagine what would have happened if that shop had called the police to handle the situation! What if the man had yelled 'Stop! Thief!!' as they used to do in the comic strips? What would have happened if, through misunderstanding of the circumstances, I had somehow ended up in court, charged with theft? My friends would have assured me of their confidence in my innocence; yet gossip would have spread the news far and wide, and subsequent acquittal would not have prevented a lingering stain of suspicion.

Some years ago, a high-profile political figure was in the news because he had been accused of stealing a box of matches from a department store. He protested that he had put the small box absent-mindedly in his pocket, intending to pay when he reached the cashier. I have forgotten the outcome, yet as a chronically absent-minded professor, I cannot forget that such a thing happened—which is why I mention so trivial an incident here. When such incidents happen (and they are not rare) the accused deserves the benefit of the doubt, not only in law, but in our mind.

What really matters

I have a dim recollection of a story about a woman on a sinking ship—one of the great luxury passenger liners. She was a very wealthy woman, and as she stood on the sloping deck waiting to be herded into one of the life-boats, she decided that there was time for her to rush back to her cabin and get something before the life-boats were lowered.

So she went back to her cabin, with its cases full of fine jewellery, its cupboards full of fine furs. And then she hurried back up to the boat deck, carrying in her hand … an orange! She knew what was important at that moment. All her splendid possessions were inconsequential.

I was reminded of this story a while ago when I suddenly realised that I had stopped doing something that I had done for years. Every year, when our family would go away on vacation, I used to hide the more portable valuables: various antique knick-nacks and things … actually, mostly my old microscopes.

I used to hide them under the beds, and behind stacks of clothes in closets and so on—not in the thought that they couldn't easily be found, but in the hope that an ordinary thief-in-a-hurry might pass them by. But somewhere along the line, without thinking much about it, I simply stopped doing this. I hope this disclosure will not put larcenous thoughts into anyone's head!

I stopped, I suppose, because deep down I must have realised that those things were absolutely inconsequential. When everyone was out of the house, everything in the house was of no consequence. Oh, there were old photographs and mementoes that would be severely missed if the house burned down, but all the 'valuables' were of no value in the larger scheme of things. In that scheme of things, people are the valuables. People are consequential. Our welfare, spiritual and material, is consequent to our interaction with people.

It is most obvious in the case of our family ties. A duty I adopted as a parent was to write a letter to each of my children when they went off to college. It is a way of marking a milestone in life's journey, although it may just reflect a compulsion to get in a final word of advice as each fledgling takes wing. My letters addressed my children as unique and beloved individuals, yet I remember a couple of things that were common to all three letters.

I urged my children to avoid a life of excessive preparation (my point above regarding preparation for public speaking not-withstanding). They would need to prepare for each step along the way, but they should resist any tendency to assume that they will really start to enjoy life, to 'live' life, once they leave college; once they get a job, or get that promotion; once they get married; once they retire … and so on. Instead, each preparatory phase should be considered a part of life, not a postponement of life. That is risky advice to give to young people, unless you know them well. It may be more useful for mature adults.

I also acknowledged that my religious faith could be described as 'fuzzy,' but made a point of telling them that, like it or not, I pray for each of my children every day of my life. I cannot know whether that has anything to do with the observable fate or welfare of the children or of others for whom I pray—for whom any of us pray. We can trust in prayer; we can mistrust; but we cannot pry deeply into prayer.

We do know that our children matter. They come under the heading of this piece simply because of who they are. It is a truism, even a tautology, to say that loved-ones matter—but I have already hinted how much Mary matters to me. The chil-dren she and I have raised seem to be forging successful paths in life. Jenifer has had a wonderful career as a school teacher of French and has become accredited as a translator; Peter is a gifted software developer; Betsy found her calling as an acupunc-turist and wellness counsellor.

They have other talents too, of course. Jenifer is a gifted artist. She is married to Andrew Bluhm, an oral surgeon, and is a key resource in the planning and implementation of meet-ings and conferences associated with his busy practice. Peter is skilled in metal-work and 3-D printing, and he makes the most wonderful toys for his nieces and nephews. I rely on him frequently and of necessity on computer-related matters; his knowledge and his patience seem equally limitless. Betsy and her husband Adam Learner brilliantly combine the deployment of their healing talents, their parenting gifts and the adminis-tration of their acupuncture and family-wellness clinic. Betsy and Jenifer are beautiful singers, as is Mary, so we know which side of the family it comes from. This was an early realisation for Betsy: 'One of my earliest memories is us being in Church as a family. My mother was typically singing in the choir and sitting close to the organ, so I would sit in the pew with my Dad. I was surprised at first when I realised he was only pretending to sing the hymns due to feeling shy about his singing voice. I felt I was let in on his little secret, and it became our little secret.' When Mary was a student at Colby College she was a member of a female chorus called the Colbyettes. I think it is wonderful that Betsy elected to go to the same university and became a member of the Colbyettes a generation after her mother.

Biased I may be, but I think that our kids are wonderful—as, too, are our five grandchildren. Two of them are launched and into adulthood now, three are still at school. Being a part of their lives is one of life's great pleasures.

One of the perils of growing older is that you lose the ones you love. My father had died in 1956, when I was still a relatively young man. My mother died in 1985. I had been at a conference in Geneva. She had been ill and while we knew the end was near, when it came it was still a shock. I immediately left the confer-ence and went to Ramelton to attend the funeral and grieve with my siblings, Bert, Lexie and Marion.

We siblings survived for many more years, keeping in touch, but that was coming to an end. In 2010, my brother Lexie died. In our childhood, Lexie had been dominating, but later in life turned out to be very caring, and when he died I felt a tremen-dous sense of loss. Years later I still miss the feeling that he is just a phone call away. Seven years later Bert, the eldest of us, was also gone, and I miss him terribly, too. His wife Anne and I remain in frequent touch by phone. I visited Bert in Ramelton in late 2017, when he was near his death. Our final evening was steeped in reminiscence. As we said goodnight, Bert in broken voice said

'I love you'. I managed to croak out those same precious words; next morning, as planned, I left before his aides had arrived to get Bert out of bed. He died less than two months later. That, I remind you, is not a tale of tearful reconciliation. The sentiment was there all along. It was the words that were missing.

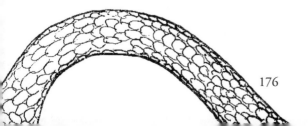

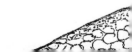

Last words

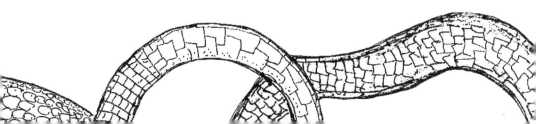

An epilogue

We live in an era of 'word processors' and torrents of words, so the writing of memoirs has become easy and popular. Composition, however, remains tricky; purpose is generally murky. It was reported that former American president Bill Clinton once blurted out his intention to write an autobiographical book. A friend said, in a voice filled with disapproval, 'But won't that be self-serving?' Clinton replied, 'I sure hope so'. Benjamin Franklin, too, embarking on his own autobiography, happily acknowledged 'perhaps I shall a good deal gratify my own vanity'. In my own defence, I must ask you, the reader, to keep in mind that while I am fully responsible for any mistakes in the present memoir, the Royal Irish Academy (see Acknowledgements) must be held accountable for its coming into existence!

I am as bereft as others of practicable solutions to the incredibly big and incredibly difficult problems that threaten the modern world. In our everyday lives, however, there are some pitfalls that might be avoided, a few conditions that might be ameliorated, by simply remaining alert.

Among the liabilities that beset us as we grow older is the tendency to be misled by our accumulated knowledge. I have known excellent scientists who, late in life, began to pontificate about which things would work, and which other things would not work. We hear more and more about people losing their creative edge in middle life. That might indeed happen; I have a suspicion that, in many cases, intellectual acumen is simply dulled by an abundance of knowledge and a loss of nerve. If we feel sure that something will not work, we will not encourage young people to do it; so young folk should listen to old folk with a sceptical ear.

From these and other experiences I am led to a conclusion that some readers might find surprising: in science, doubt is our stoutest ally. Oddly enough, doubt is central to both science and religion—for science contends with doubt, and faith is meaningful only in the context of doubt.

I have suggested elsewhere that the initial negative reaction to the report of ivermectin's potential utility (in controlling river blindness) might have been an example of experts being victimised by their own expertise. Another example might be more instructive: I knew a distinguished academic scientist, a member of a governmental review panel, who rejected a research proposal that was very much in his area of science, and which was designed to test a simple hypothesis. His stated reason for rejecting the proposal was that if the hypothesis were to be supported by experimentation, the level of science in that area was not sufficiently advanced to enable interpretation of the result. That reflects a bizarre blindness to the reality of science. I have no doubt that validation of the hypothesis would, in itself, have provided a new tool—one that could be used to advance the science.

My life has been long in years, and rich in good fortune. Chance plays a big part in most lives. (I try to avoid the word luck; it smacks a little of the roulette wheel and the crapshoot.) Chance can bring us bad fortune as well as good. One can view chance as random; or one can attribute it to something ineffable, something beyond the reach of human understanding. Either way, our challenge is to use it constructively.

Most of us have been born into love. Most of us have experienced the giving and receiving of love in our lives. For some, the experience has been, or has seemed to have been, tragically deficient or even lacking. I have been fortunate and am correspondingly grateful; although the match is not over, I hope someday to echo my father's last words: 'I have had a good innings'.

ACKNOWLEDGEMENTS

Gratitude toward family and intimate friends is a sentiment that is light-years beyond any capacity of mere words to encompass. Many of those individuals will have cameo roles in the present production; but they and their off-stage colleagues will know full well the depth of my love, and the reality of my indebtedness to them.

I am forever grateful to Merck & Co. Inc. for employing me for 33 years, and sustaining me through times when I found it hard to believe that they were paying me for having fun doing research on worm disease, and times when I resorted to serious consideration of other employment. Desmond Smyth, my mentor at Trinity College Dublin, imparted fascination and gave direction to my life's work.

I am more grateful than I can say to Drew University for giving to me, and to many others, a unique opportunity to repay a mentor by becoming a mentor. Thanks to the efforts of its trustees, faculty, and the Research Institute for Scientists Emeriti, countless 'out-to-pasture' retirement hours have been converted into an investment in the life potential of those who follow us.

$\sim$

I have always enjoyed writing, so it is not surprising that in old age I was in the habit of jotting down brief memoirs on a wide variety of topics. Beneath it all, there was a vague sense that—'someday'—I would pull those pieces together in book form. That gave way to a stronger suspicion that, given how busy I was in old age, and given my proclivity for putting things off, I was unlikely to live long enough, or to become motivated enough, for a book to materialise. That is where the Royal Irish Academy stepped in.

Its president Peter Kennedy wrote to inquire whether I might be interested in collaboration with the Academy in the way of pulling memoirs together, expediting their creation, or in some other way getting the story of my life and work down on paper. Thus began a collaboration for which I here express my profound thanks to Professor Kennedy.

The Academy's managing editor Ruth Hegarty and head of public affairs Pauric Dempsey, working in collaboration with journalist-scientist Claire O'Connell have brought this book into being. The text has benefited enormously from the insights of early reviewers—to whom we owe many thanks—and from the brilliant editing of Helena King. The book was designed by Fidelma Slattery, and her superb artistry is right here for all to see. The process of creation was intense. The declaration that 'failure is not an option' became something of a cliché in the world of space travel; in the present case, procrastination was not an option. That reality presented an ongoing challenge, for we all had other things to do. I am immensely grateful to Ruth Hegarty—and indeed the entire Publications Office team of the Royal Irish Academy—for bringing our endeavour to a successful conclusion.

It is a special pleasure to record my deep thanks to Claire O'Connell. She worked tirelessly to get to know me and my work personally and professionally. Above all, she respected my selfish desire to let my writings remain (for better or for worse) in 'my voice'. It was not always easy to reconcile that desire with her goal of knitting my fragments together, transplanting topics and adding 'connective tissue' to fill in gaps in the narrative. Claire talked at length to my wife Mary and me about family and work. From those sessions, we derived much enjoyment and she derived the information and perspective needed for her writing. Most significantly, Claire has introduced a chronological structure and has given an overall coherence to the book.

∿

Because of my preoccupation with the book, my family and friends, and especially my wife Mary, have had to put up with much. Members of devoted families do willingly put up with much. We should be grateful, and I believe we are.

I have dedicated this book not only to family and friends, but to former colleagues. I trust that my colleagues will understand that those words of dedication convey my most profound respect, admiration and gratitude.

WCC. March 2020

SELECT BIBLIOGRAPHY

Thomas Kingsmill Abbott 1900 *The elements of logic* (4th edn). Dublin. Hodges, Figgis.

Ellen Agler 2019 *Under the big tree*. Baltimore, MD. Johns Hopkins University Press.

Bruce Benton 2020 (forthcoming) *Riverblindness in Africa— taming the lion's stare*. Baltimore, MD. Johns Hopkins University Press.

Francisco Battistini 1969 'Treatment of creeping eruption with topical thiabendazole', *Texas Reports on Biology and Medicine* 27 (supplement 2) (November), 645–58.

William C. Campbell 1983 *Trichinella and trichinosis*. New York and London. Plenum Press.

William C. Campbell 1988a, 1988b, 1990 Poems, *Perspectives in Biology and Medicine*: 'Fasciola', 31 (4), 506; 'Onchocerca', 32 (1), 108; 'M & B 693', 33 (3), 389–90.

William C. Campbell 2012 'History of ivermectin and abamectin: with notes on the history of later macrocyclic lactone antiparasitic agents', *Current Pharmacology and Biotechnology* 13, 853–65.

William C. Campbell 2016 'Point of clarification', Letters, *Irish America* (October/November), 8; available online at: https://irishamerica.com/archives/2016-archive/october-november -2016/.

Brenda Colatrella 2008 'The Mectizan Donation Program: 20 years of successful collaboration', *Annals of Tropical Medicine and Parasitology* 102 (Suppl. 1), 7–11.

Heinz Goerke 1973 *Linnaeus*. New York. Scribner.

Patricia Harty 2016 'A reflection on simplicity', *Irish America* (August/September), 28–32 and 88; available online at: https://irishamerica.com/2016/08/a-reflection-on-simplicity/.

William Kirby 1835 *On the history, habits and instincts of animals* (2 vols). The Bridgewater Treatises: Treatise VII. London. William Pickering.

Alan Lightman 2018 *Searching for stars on an island in Maine*. New York. Pantheon Books.

Arthur Mee (ed.) 1910 *The children's encyclopaedia*. London. Educational Book Company.

James Pope-Hennessy 1971 *Anthony Trollope*. London. Jonathan Cape.

Thomas Sprat 1667 *The history of the Royal Society of London for the improving of natural knowledge*. London. T.R. for J. Martyn, and J. Allestry.

Anthony Trollope 1883 *An autobiography of Anthony Trollope*. Edinburgh and London. William Blackwood and Sons.

David Allardice Webb 1943 *An Irish flora*. Dundalk. Dundalgan Press.

Index

72
79   98
p·110
116
136
150